Medicines Management
for Nursing Practice

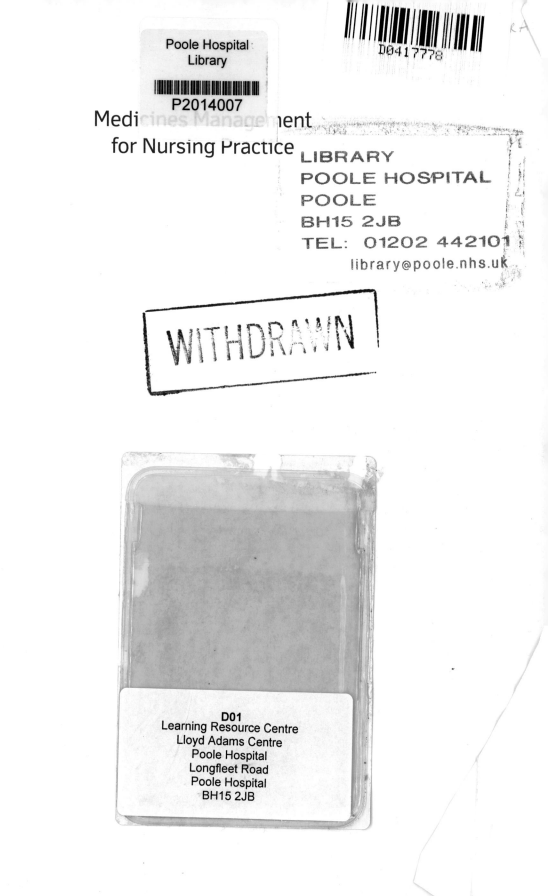

Medicines Management for Nursing Practice

Pharmacology, patient safety, and procedures

Graham Brack
Plymouth University

Penny Franklin
Plymouth University

Jill Caldwell
Oxford Brookes University

With contributions from

Mark Wilbourn
University of Western Sydney

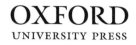

OXFORD
UNIVERSITY PRESS

OXFORD
UNIVERSITY PRESS

Great Clarendon Street, Oxford OX2 6DP,
United Kingdom

Oxford University Press is a department of the University of Oxford.
It furthers the University's objective of excellence in research, scholarship,
and education by publishing worldwide. Oxford is a registered trade mark of
Oxford University Press in the UK and in certain other countries

British Library Cataloguing in Publication Data
Data available

ISBN 978-0-19-969787-8

Printed in Great Britain by
Ashford Colour Press Ltd, Gosport, Hampshire

Foreword

The use of medicines in the UK is sub-optimal. Research evidence indicates that patients are sometimes harmed from preventable medication errors, the most effective medicines are not always selected, health professionals and patients do not always use medicines as intended and too many medicines are wasted.

In a review of over 500,000 medication incidents reported to the National Reporting and Learning System in England and Wales between 2005–2010 the top three types of incidents concerned omitted and delayed medicines, wrong dose, and wrong medicine (Cousins et al, 2012). Groups of medicines most commonly involved in incidents leading to death and severe harm were Controlled Drugs (opioids and benzodiazepines), antibiotics, anticoagulants (warfarin and low molecular weight heparin), insulin and non-steroidal anti-inflammatory drugs (Cousins et al, 2012).

These incidents result from problems in practice, the design of medicine products, medical devices, procedures and healthcare systems. Patient safety improvements demand a complex system-wide effort, involving patients, carers, health professionals, health providers, health commissioners, regulators and industry.

Nurses are the most numerous of the healthcare professions and a significant percentage of their professional practice involves the use of medicines .Improving knowledge, understanding and practice of nurses on the safe and effective use of medicines will help to minimise harms and optimise the use of medicines. Nurses have an individual professional responsibility to promote safer medicines practice, but it is particularly important that nurses also understand and promote the need for safe medication systems. The safe use of medicines is everybody's business. I welcome this medicines management publication for nurses that provides comprehensive information on best practice, science and regulation of medicines.

Dr David Cousins

Associate Director – Safe Medication Practice and Medical Devices

NHS Commissioning Board

Reference

Cousins D, Gerrett D, Warner B (2012) Reporting and Learning System in England and Wales over six years (2005– 2010) *Br J Clin Pharmacol*. 74: 597–604

Preface

This book is designed to provide an overview of the issues and knowledge required to provide safe and effective medicines management to patients. In the first chapter student nurses will find details of the Nursing and Midwifery Council's essential skills cluster related to medicines management, and can identify where within the book they will find the relevant information for each outcome. The book is not intended to explore specific fields of nursing in any depth but is about medicines management generally. Although we have used the term 'medicines management' throughout, there is a movement towards using 'medicines optimization', which is seen as a more patient-centred expression.

Use of the term 'nurse' acknowledges that those reading this book may be student nurses or registered practitioners. Students may not be involved in some of the scenarios discussed but they may want to discuss with their mentors how these may need to be dealt with.

A nurse who is working in the adult field will be caring for a large number of older people. As people age their major organs are prone to deteriorate; it is important for nurses to be aware of how deterioration in liver and kidney function can change the metabolism of drugs in older patients. Similarly, younger patients might also have specific organ dysfunction and this will affect their processing of medicines and how the medicines work in their body. These issues are important to take into account but are not covered in depth within this book.

The layout of the book allows readers to select individual chapters and references are made to where other relevant issues are covered. All chapters have clear learning outcomes and activities such as reflection on aspects of practice. References are identified at the end of each chapter.

We hope you find this book interesting and easy to use. The aim is to encourage all nurses to understand the important factors that will ensure they manage medicines in a safe and effective manner and that patients will gain maximum benefit from their medicines.

Table of Contents

About the authors   xiii

List of Abbreviations   xiv

How to use this book   xv

1 Legislation and Standards   1

2 Patient Safety and Error Reduction   25

3 Principles of Pharmacology   42

4 Pharmaceutics and Routes of Drug Administration   70

5 Groups at Special Risk of Adverse Effects   82

6 Information and Evidence: Sources and Evaluation   98

7 Medicines Management: Systems and Procedures   108

8 Medicines Management: Drug Calculations   126

9 The Nurse's Role in Promoting Concordance   133

10 Keeping Up to Date   144

Glossary   157

Index   159

Detailed Contents

About the authors   xiii
List of Abbreviations   xiv
How to use this book   xv

| Chapter 1 **Legislation and Standards** | 1 |

Introduction   1
Accountability and responsibility   2
Legislation   3
The legal roles of various health professionals   7
Who can administer drugs?   10
Prescriptions   11
Patient group directions and patient specific directions   11
Quiz   16
Patients and their legal rights   17
What nurses need to know about medicines management   20
Summary   23

| Chapter 2 **Patient Safety and Error Reduction** | 25 |

How can we reduce the incidence of harm from medication?   27
The importance of near misses   27
Never events   28
What actions most commonly lead to mistakes?   28
Reason's Swiss cheese model of errors   32
Active failures and latent conditions   35
The system approach in action   35
Using guidelines and protocols to reduce risks   36
Learning from our mistakes   38
Serious untoward incident policies   38
The national reporting and learning system (NRLS)
and the yellow card system   39
Personal accountability   39
Summary   40

Chapter 3 Principles of Pharmacology   42

Basic pharmacokinetics   43
Absorption   44
Distribution   48
Metabolism   51
Excretion   55
Key pharmacokinetic concepts   56
Pharmacogenetics   57
Pharmacodynamics   58
Adverse drug reactions   63
Drug interactions   65
Quiz   65
Complementary medicines   67
Summary   67

Chapter 4 Pharmaceutics and Routes of Drug Administration   70

Routes of administration: pros and cons   70
Oral administration   71
Enteral administration   73
Rectal and vaginal routes   74
Respiratory route   74
Injections and infusions   75
Topical or transdermal   79
Summary   81

Chapter 5 Groups at Special Risk of Adverse Effects   82

Groups of patients who are at special risk   82
Circumstances that might pose a risk to patients   83
The older patient   84
Medicines and patients who have hepatic impairment   88
Medicines and patients who have renal impairment   88
Medicines and the pregnant woman   88
Medicines and women who are breastfeeding   89
Medicines and children   90
Medicines and patients with cognitive impairment and learning disability   93
Polypharmacy: the nurse and the patient   94
Summary   96

Chapter 6 **Information and Evidence: Sources and Evaluation**   98

Information sources   98
Assessing, critiquing, and critical appraisal   102
The British National Formulary (BNF)   103
Understanding evaluations   105
Summary   106

Chapter 7 **Medicines Management: Systems and Procedures**   108

Why do we need systems and procedures?   109
Medicines management: definitions   109
Components of medicines management   110
Standards for medicines management   111
Responsibility   112
Accountability   112
Stock management   114
One stop dispensing   115
Reducing risk by proper organization of stock cupboards and drug trolleys   115
Medicines administration records and record keeping   116
What is medicines reconciliation?   119
Taking a medicines history on admission: the acquisition
of necessary practical skills   119
Quiz   120
National standards for medicines management   121
The role of the Care Quality Commission   122
Summary   123

Chapter 8 **Medicines Management: Drug Calculations**   126

Introduction to drug calculations   126
SI units   127
How to convert metric units   127
Calculating drug dosages   128
Weight-related doses   131
Summary   132

Chapter 9 **The Nurse's Role in Promoting Concordance**   133

Compliance versus adherence and concordance   133
Things that can go wrong with medication   134
Concordance   134
Patient health: beliefs and concordance   134
Adherence   136

Adverse drug reactions and concordance   137
Patients posing particular difficulty   138
Preparing a patient for discharge   140
Expert patient programme   141
Summary   142

Chapter 10 **Keeping Up to Date**   144

Introduction   144
New roles and organizations   146
Medicines and change management   146
Working with others   148
Clinical governance and patient safety   148
Clinical audit   149
Risk management   150
Workforce issues   151
Clinical supervision   152
Competencies and revalidation   152
Delegation   153
Specialized skills for particular settings   154
Summary   154

Glossary   157
Index   159

About the authors

Graham Brack is a community pharmacist in Cornwall who also holds appointments as Pharmaceutical Adviser for Cornwall & Isles of Scilly Primary Care Trust and as an Associate Lecturer in Pharmacology for the University of Plymouth. He is a member of the Editorial Board of the journal Pharmacy Management and is a frequent contributor to its pages. He holds a Master's degree in medical law and ethics and was a member of the NICE/National Patient Safety Agency joint committee on medicines reconciliation safety, and was a member of the Department of Health's Controlled Drugs Action Group. He is himself an independent prescriber specializing in the care of substance misusers and has been involved in teaching nurse prescribers since the very first cohort in Cornwall.

Penny Franklin is a Senior Lecturer at the University of Plymouth where she leads the programme for Non-medical Prescribing and is a co-author of the Oxford Handbook of Prescribing for Nurses and Allied Health Professionals. She also teaches medication management to pre and post qualifying nurses. Penny is a Registered General Nurse, Registered Children's Nurse, and Registered Community Specialist Public Health Nurse (Health Visitor) and engages in public health practice on a regular basis. In addition she is a Registered Nurse Teacher and a Community Practitioner Nurse Prescriber and Nurse Independent and Supplementary Prescriber. Penny has strong links with organizational Non-medical Leads locally and nationally. Penny holds a Masters of Arts (with distinction) in Complementary Health Studies and a Post Graduate Certificate in Health Care and Higher Education (LTHE). She is a Fellow of the Institute of Teaching and Learning in Higher Education.

Jill Caldwell is a Senior Lecturer in the Faculty of Health and Life Sciences at Oxford Brookes University. She has a BSc in Community Health Care and a Masters in Higher Professional Education and has been teaching both undergraduate and postgraduate nursing students for 10 years. During this time she has also been involved in teaching on the Non-Medical Prescribing course offered at Oxford Brookes University.

List of Abbreviations

ARR	absolute risk reduction	NPC	National Prescribing Centre
AO	accountable officer	NRLS	National Reporting and Learning System
ADR	adverse drug reaction		
ACE	angiotensin converting enzyme	NETSCC	NIHR Evaluation, Trials, and Studies Coordinating Centre
BNFC	BNF for Children		
BNF	*British National Formulary*	NSAID	non-steroidal anti-inflammatory drug
CQC	Care Quality Commission	NNH	number needed to harm
CMP	clinical management plan	NNT	number needed to treat
CSCI	Commission for Social Care Inspection	NMC	Nursing and Midwifery Council
CPD	continuing professional development	OTIS	Organization of Teratology Information Specialists
CDRC	controlled drugs record card		
CASP	critical appraisal skills programme	OTC	over the counter
DH	Department of Health	PIP	paediatric investigation plan
DTB	Drug and Therapeutics Bulletin	PUMA	paediatric use marketing authorization
FTU	fingertip unit	PGD	patienl group direction
GMC	General Medical Council	PSD	patient specific direction
GSL	general sales list	POD	patients own drugs
GFR	glomerular filtration rate	PACT	prescribing analysis and cost tool
HPC	Health Professions Council	POM	prescription-only medicine
HTA	health technology assessment	PCT	primary care trust
IHI	Institute for Healthcare Improvement	RRR	relative risk reductions
ICMJE	International Committee of Medical Journal Editors	RPSGB	Royal Pharmaceutical Society for Great Britain (now the Royal Pharmaceutical Society (RPS))
LPA	lasting power of attorney		
LIN	local intelligence network	SIGN	Scottish Intercollegiate Guidelines Network
MUST	malnutrition universal screening tool		
MAR	medicines administration record	SSRI	selective serotonin re-uptake inhibitor
MHRA	Medicines and Healthcare products Regulatory Agency	SUI	serious untoward incidents
		SEA	significant event analysis
MDS	monitored dosage system	SOP	standard operating procedures
MAOI	monoamine oxidase inhibitor	CRD	The Centre for Reviews and Dissemination
MDT	multidisciplinary team		
NaDIA	National Diabetes Inpatient Audits	UKMi	United Kingdom Medicines Information
NICE	National Institute for Health and Clinical Excellence	VAD	vascular access device
		VGCC	voltage-gated calcium channel
NIHR	National Institute for Health Research	WAME	World Association of Medical Editors
NPSA	National Patient Safety Agency		

How to use this book

Medicines Management for Nursing Practice explains how to manage and administer medications in a safe, patient-centred way. This brief tour of the book shows you how to get the most out of this textbook.

Finding your way through

Find what you need fast The detailed list of contents in the front of the book and the list of learning objectives at the beginning of each chapter will help you navigate this book.

What does that mean? New terms are highlighted in bold in the text – go to the glossary at the back of the book to see their definitions.

> The results of clinical trials may also be expressed as **risk reductions**. Drug companies often want to promote their drugs using **relative risk reductions (RRR)**. These make the effect of the drug look much more impressive, but may be misleading if the event

Bringing theory to life

Numbered boxes highlight extra information to help you take your understanding further.

> **Box 7.1** Safely storing medicines
>
> - Are they stored in a safe place?
> - Are they stored at the correct temperature?
> - Who has access to the stored medicines?

Exercises and Activities help you to test your knowledge and put theory into real-world situations.

> **Exercise 8.2 Calculating liquid drug dosages**
>
> Now try calculating this one on your own: if there is 40 mg of the drug in 5 mL what is the amount you would need to administer to give a dose of 20 mg?

Case studies present you with situations you're likely to encounter as a qualified nurse and help you plan how you might react.

> **Case study 9.1**
>
> Mrs Khan is a widow in her seventies. She came to the United Kingdom in her middle age and has never mastered English, but within her community this has

Reflection points give you a chance to reflect on situations you've experienced in the past, and how you might learn from them to improve your practice.

> **Reflection point**
>
> Reflect on your experiences of supporting patients with difficulties.
> What factors did you need to consider?

Next steps

Conclusions at the end of every chapter summarise what has been covered and give you the opportunity to assess your progress.

Summary

This chapter explored the theory of concordance and has provided a range of information to enable you to understand the concept. It has also detailed some

Further reading lists direct you to the best sources of evidence and information for more in-depth study.

Further reading

Students who wish to develop their knowledge of pharmacokinetics further may find *Clinical Pharmacokinetics* by Dhillon and Kostrzewski (2006) useful. Appendix 1 of the *BNF* contains many drug interactions, though it

1 Legislation and Standards

CHAPTER CONTENTS

- Introduction
- Accountability and responsibility
- Legislation
- The legal roles of various health professionals
- Who can administer drugs?
- Prescriptions
- Patient group directions and patient specific directions
- Quiz
- Patients and their legal rights
- What nurses need to know about medicines management
- Summary

LEARNING OUTCOMES

- To look at the legal, professional, and clinical boundaries relating to accountability and responsibility and apply these in relation to the administration and supply of medicines
- To examine the implications of these boundaries in relation to individual practice
- To understand the major legislation relating to medicines
- To distinguish between the Medicines Act and the Misuse of Drugs Act
- To understand the changes in the use of controlled drugs brought about by the Shipman Inquiry
- To understand which nurses can prescribe and how
- To understand when a student nurse can administer medicines and how this should be undertaken
- To understand the terms 'patient group directions' and 'patient specific directions' and interpret their relevance to the prescribing, administration, and supply of medicines.

Introduction

Handling medicines is only part of the nurse's role, but it is a very important part. Handled properly, medicines can make a great contribution to improving the health of your patients. Handled badly, they can do a lot of harm. It is therefore not surprising that there is a lot of legislation relating to medicines, and that the Nursing and Midwifery Council has laid down important standards for the way in which nurses conduct the management of medicines.

The legislation is complex, but it has to be learned. Nurses do not need to become lawyers, but they do need a working knowledge of the law relating to medicines so that they can keep within it. This chapter will set out some of the key legislation that will affect your practice as a student or qualified nurse. It will also look at the rights that patients have and give you the opportunity to reflect on the practice you see around you. Most of us will be patients ourselves at some time and we will have a good idea of the way in which we would want to be treated by nurses. It is too easy for people who care for others to fall into the trap of doing what they think is best for the patient, or for their own good, and ignoring the patient's legitimate wishes. After reading this chapter, you should know how this can be avoided.

You cannot register as a nurse without demonstrating knowledge of medicines management. Understanding the laws and regulations that are relevant is the first step in building that knowledge. The law on medicines is primarily designed to keep patients safe, so a nurse who does not know it is unlikely to be able to practise safely. As was remarked in the foreword, the main aim of this book is to help you do that.

Accountability and responsibility

The concepts of accountability and responsibility are fundamental to any practice related to the administration of medicines. They are inter-related but distinct.

Accountability involves being called to explain (account for) your actions or omissions by someone to whom you owe a duty. This might be a legal duty, a professional duty, a contractual duty, or a civil duty arising from a duty of care. Nurses are therefore accountable to a range of others.

Exercise 1.1

Reflect for a few moments on those to whom you are accountable for the care you give. Make a list and compare it with ours.

You may be accountable to:

- Society in general, which is done through the criminal law. If you break the law, you can be prosecuted

- Your professional body—the Nursing and Midwifery Council (NMC) or the Health Professions Council (HPC)—for practice that does not meet their standards

- Your employer, because your contract of employment will set out the duties you have and failure to meet those may result in disciplinary action

- Your patients, who can use the civil law to sue you (or your employers) if your care falls short of the standard that they are entitled to expect.

Some people would add that you are accountable to yourself too, because good practitioners who take reflective practice seriously will set themselves high standards.

Your accountability is personal, and you cannot shelter behind anyone else. It is possible for more than one person to be accountable for an episode of care. We are all accountable for what we do, seen in the light of what can reasonably be expected of us. As a student, you may not have the experience or knowledge to undertake a task, but you discharge your accountability by making that clear to anyone who attempts to delegate that task to you. That person has their own accountability, which involves not delegating work to someone who cannot complete it.

Current NMC Guidance for Nursing and Midwifery Students (NMC, 2009a) enshrines four core principles which are relevant here:

- Make the care of people your first concern, treating them as individuals and respecting their dignity

- Work with others to protect and promote the health and wellbeing of those in your care, families and carers, and the wider community

- Provide a high standard of practice and care at all times

- Be open and honest, act with integrity, and uphold the reputation of your profession.

Accountability describes how we relate to others for what we do. Responsibility describes our sense of ownership for the quality of the tasks that make up the care we provide. We are responsible for all that we do (or fail to do) when we provide care. Even if we were not accountable to anyone else, we would still be responsible for what we did, and good reflective practice should make clear to us what standards we expect ourselves to meet. Responsibility will also include a duty to improve our practice by seeking help from those who can assist us. Seen in this way, our 'accountability' to ourselves is probably better seen as a responsibility to be the best practitioner that we can be.

Legislation

In January 2010, the Government issued an apology to families affected by the use of the drug thalidomide (Bosely, 2010). Between 1959 and 1962, thalidomide was widely prescribed as a sleeping tablet. During this time it was noted that an unusual number of babies were being born with major limb deformities. This condition (called phocomelia, because the babies' arms or legs resembled seals' flippers) is very rarely seen, but before long many obstetricians were reporting that they had seen such a case. Evidence accumulated that suggested that thalidomide given to women in the first trimester of pregnancy was the likeliest cause. At that time, a manufacturer could introduce a medicine to the market with very few restrictions. If the medicine was sold, the Sale of Goods Act applied, and it had to be fit for the purpose for which it was sold, but a prescription medicine is not 'sold', so the legislation was unlikely to be helpful to someone who had been damaged. Following the thalidomide tragedy, the law relating to medicines, their sale, and supply was considerably revised. The result was the Medicines Act (1968), which, in conjunction with some European legislation, now governs the supply of medicinal products in the United Kingdom.

The term '**medicinal product**' is used rather than 'medicine' in the legislation. According to European Council Directive 2004/27/EC, an item is a medicinal product if it is presented as having properties for treating or preventing disease in human beings. This means that alternative medicines and health foods may be included if therapeutic claims are made for them. For example, it is often claimed that an herbal product can boost one's immune system. Whether there is evidence

for this or not, the fact that the claim is made will make that product a medicinal product. It is important to note that it is not the drug that is classified in this way, but the product. If company A claims that their product prevents the common cold, while company B does not, then A's product is a medicinal product while B's will not be. A real-life example can be seen when comparing products for hyperhidrosis (excessive sweating). These are more powerful versions of standard antiperspirants, but some are designed to treat this medical condition and are therefore medicinal products, while other products, made to an identical recipe, are not advertised for the prevention of excessive sweating and are marketed as cosmetics. Since the medicinal product will have undergone some testing, while the cosmetic may not have done, we are required to use the licensed medicinal product whenever possible.

An additional, wider definition is given in the same directive:

> **A substance or combination of substances which may be used in or administered to human beings either with a view to restoring, correcting or modifying physiological functions by exerting a pharmacological, immunological or metabolic action or to making a medical diagnosis**
> European Council Directive 2004/27/EC

The Council directive also covers the possibility that a product may be a medicinal product and also defined as something else such as a health food. In such circumstances, the product must be treated as a medicinal product even if the manufacturer describes it in other terms.

The Medicines Act 1968

Before a medicinal product can be sold or supplied in the United Kingdom, it must have a **marketing authorization** (previously known as a product licence) or meet one of a list of specified exemptions, such as being prepared for an individual patient according to a formula supplied by a suitable practitioner. Each stage of the manufacturing, importing, and distribution process is subject to licensing arrangements administered by the Medicines and Healthcare products Regulatory Authority (MHRA).

The marketing authorization specifies the uses for which the medicinal product is licensed. For example, it may be licensed for the treatment of angina in adults. As more evidence becomes available, the makers can submit evidence to MHRA and ask for new **indications** to be added to the authorization. If a product does not have a marketing authorization of any kind, it is described an **unlicensed**. If it is used outside the terms of its authorization, it is described as off-licence or off-label. This is an important distinction as we shall see later.

One of the most common restrictions on the use of a medicinal product is the specification of a minimum age for use. This means that many well-known medicines are not licensed for paediatric use. Aspirin, for example, cannot generally be used in those under 16 years of age because it can cause Reye's syndrome, a rare but dangerous condition (Joint Formulary Committee, BNF, hardcopy updated six-monthly). However, there are some circumstances in which specialists may decide it is the best treatment for a child under their care, based upon their experience and their knowledge of the evidence available. Prescribers who wish to use unlicensed medicines, or licensed medicines outside the terms of their licence, therefore do so under their own responsibility. This will be discussed in more detail in Chapter 4.

The Medicines Act (1968) divided medicinal products into three groups for the purposes of restricting their sale or supply. The default position is that medicinal products should only be sold under the supervision of a pharmacist. Such 'pharmacy-only medicines' are marked on the original container with a letter P inside a box, thus: P.

Products which are regarded as safe enough for no such restriction to be necessary are included on a general sales list (GSL). There is no marking on the package, but some formularies or suppliers' lists denote these with the abbreviation GSL. It is important to note that the designation relates to the particular product and pack listed. Larger packs may not be on the GSL list. For example, paracetamol 500mg tablets are on the GSL in pack sizes up to 16 tablets. Packs up to 32 are pharmacy-only medicines, and larger packs than these are prescription-only.

Prescription-only medicines (POM) are marked POM on the original container. As the name implies, they may only be supplied by authorized persons such as pharmacists and dispensing doctors in accordance with a practitioner's prescription, though others may be authorized to use them in their professional practice.

The Misuse of Drugs Act 1971

Readers of the Sherlock Holmes detective stories may recall that Holmes was a regular user of injected cocaine. At the time that the stories were written, from 1891 onwards, there were few restrictions on the supply of cocaine, and Holmes would have had little difficulty in obtaining a quantity for personal use. The Pharmacy Act of 1868 placed restrictions on supply of opium and its preparations and empowered the Pharmaceutical Society of Great Britain to declare items to be poisons (Pharmacy Act 1868, ss.2 and 15). This power was used in 1906 to restrict sales of any solution containing more than 1% opium. The International Opium Convention at The Hague in 1911–12 produced international agreement on restricting the trade in opium, with each signatory being required to make the necessary changes in its own laws to restrict opioids to medical uses only (League of Nations (1922)). The coming of the First World War stalled these changes, but the Convention agreement was incorporated as Article 295 of the Treaty of Versailles (HMSO, 1919) at the end of the war. (Box 1.1 gives more information on the early use of stimulants in soft drinks.)

The United Kingdom had already made temporary regulations in 1916 under the Defence of the Realm Act (1914) which made possession or supply of opium, cocaine, and morphine subject to regulation by the Home Office. These regulations lapsed at the end of the war, but were then reimposed under the Dangerous Drugs Act (1920). With various amendments, this legislation remained in force until 1967, at which point a new Dangerous Drugs Act (1967) was introduced which restricted prescribing for addicts to specialists and increased the penalties for improper use.

Following the introduction of the Medicines Act (1968), the Dangerous Drugs Act needed revision to reflect the new legal framework. The Misuse of Drugs

Box 1.1 Opiates and soft drinks

In 1885 the pharmacist John Pemberton, who practised in Atlanta, Georgia, devised a new patent medicine which he called 'Pemberton's French coca wine' (Streatfeild, 2003). It contained cocaine mixed in wine and was sold as a stimulant. Soon afterwards a new state law meant that the alcohol had to be omitted, so Pemberton changed his formula and dissolved the cocaine in flavoured carbonated water. It was sold in drugstores from soda fountains, and Pemberton claimed that it would cure a wide range of diseases, including indigestion, headache, and sexual impotence. Since it no longer contained wine,

he changed its name to Coca-Cola, because it contained cocaine and kola nuts. While he kept the formula secret, it is thought that it may have contained up to nine milligrams of cocaine in each glass.

Concerns about addiction to cocaine, and the success of competitors that contained less cocaine, led to the removal of cocaine from the formula in 1903. It is believed that coca leaves are still involved in the manufacture of Coca-Cola™ but only after all the cocaine has been removed (Pendergrast, 2000).

Act (1971) which replaced it divided dangerous drugs into schedules and classes. The schedules have implications for how these medicines are prescribed, stored, or supplied, and are numbered 1–5. The classes, A, B, and C relate to the penalties to be imposed for illegal use. Thus, the painkiller diamorphine (also known as heroin) is in schedule 2 and class A, while diazepam, which may be used a sedative or to treat anxiety, is in schedule 4, part 1, and is a class C drug. There has been much controversy about the placing of particular drugs such as ecstasy and cannabis in classes A, B, or C. In 2009 a leading member of the Advisory Council on the Misuse of Drugs, Professor David Nutt, was asked to resign because he disagreed with the decision that the UK government had taken on the classification of cannabis (Brown, 2009). However, the division of drugs into the various schedules is generally uncontroversial. While new drugs are occasionally added to the schedules, it is very unusual for them to be moved between them.

The practical implications of the schedules in the Misuse of Drugs Act (1971) are given in Table 1.1.

Changes arising from the Shipman Inquiry

Dr Harold Shipman was a general practitioner in Greater Manchester who was found guilty in 2000 of murdering 15 patients, though the subsequent public inquiry, the Shipman Inquiry, suggested that his real number of victims may have been about 250. The

reports of the Shipman Inquiry can be seen at **http://www.shipman-inquiry.org.uk/reports.asp**.

These reports were published at intervals between 2002 and 2005.

He used opiate drugs to kill his patients, and was able to obtain these, despite the regulations then in force, by diverting stocks intended for other patients. In some cases he collected unused ampoules when a patient died, and in others he ordered large quantities for a patient and collected them himself, so that he was able to remove some before the patient received them. The Shipman Inquiry produced a large number of recommendations for changes in law and practice to reduce the risk of a recurrence. It is important to note that it was widely accepted that complete security could only be achieved by introducing rules so restrictive that patient care would suffer, and therefore the remit of the inquiry was to produce recommendations that were practical and did not have an adverse effect on patients.

The Shipman Inquiry made a number of recommendations for improving the training of coroners, tightening procedures for the authorization of cremations, and changing the workings of the General Medical Council (GMC). Although the GMC had been aware of relevant incidents in Dr Shipman's past, there had been no obligation to share these, even in the public interest (Smith, 2004).

Organizations in which controlled drugs are used are now placed under an obligation to exchange information about matters of concern so that data about an

Table 1.1 Practical implications of the schedules in the Misuse of Drugs Act (1971): Guide for possession and supply of controlled drugs.

Drug schedule	Schedule 2		Schedule 3						Schedule 4	Schedule 5
	General	Secobarbital	General	Phenobarbital	Temazepam	Diethylpropion, Flunitrazepam	Buprenorphine	Midazolam		
Prescription requirements (words/figures etc.)	Yes	Yes	Yes	Yes	No	Yes	Yes	Yes	No	No
Handwriting requirements	Handwritten prescriptions are no longer necessary for any CD									
Requisitions necessary for 'bag stock'	Yes	Yes	Yes	Yes	Yes	Yes	Yes	Yes	No	No
Records of stock and use to be kept in a CD register	Yes	Yes	No	No	No	No	No	No	No	No
Emergency supplies allowed from pharmacies	No	No	No	Yes	No	No	No	No	Yes	Yes
Store in a locked receptacle	Yes	No	No	No	Yes	Yes	Yes	No	No	No
Date of supply to be marked on NHS prescription	Yes	Yes	Yes	Yes	Yes	Yes	Yes	Yes	No	No
'CD' endorsement on NHS prescriptions	No	No	No	No	No	No	No	No	No	No
Stock destruction to be witnessed	Yes	Yes	No	No	No	No	No	No	No	No
Validity of prescription	28 days	28 days	28 days	28 days	28 days	28 days	28 days	28 days	28 days	6 months
Invoices to be kept for 2 years	No	No	Yes	Yes	Yes	Yes	Yes	Yes	No	Yes

individual can be brought together. This is achieved through local intelligence networks (LINs) led by Primary Care Trusts (PCTs) or their equivalent. These LINs may cover more than one PCT by agreement, and must meet quarterly. Formal reports are made by healthcare providers who make up the network relating to the organization's use of controlled drugs. For example,

significant untoward incidents are shared so that all organizations can learn from them.

Each organization is required to appoint an Accountable Officer for controlled drugs. There is a specification for the role which explains the characteristics of the person, one of which is that they must not ordinarily handle or use controlled drugs in their professional work. Thus, a Director of Nursing may be suitable, whereas a nurse who still carries a caseload would not be. The Accountable Officer reports to their organization's board or similar supervisory body, and can appoint suitable persons to witness the destruction of controlled drugs in their district or Trust. By increasing the number of witnesses it is hoped that destruction of unwanted controlled drugs will be timelier.

Private prescribing and requisition of controlled drugs is now monitored by PCTs and the Prescription Pricing Division of the NHS Business Services Authority, for which purpose pharmacists submit the specified forms that must now be used to obtain stocks.

A key recommendation of the Shipman Inquiry which has not been implemented at the time of writing is the Controlled Drugs Record Card (CDRC). This document will be generated when injectable schedule 2 controlled drugs are dispensed for use in the community and will indicate the quantity supplied. It is a self-carboned document, one part of which is sent directly to the PCT, thus ensuring that a record exists of the amount originally dispensed. At the end of treatment the last healthcare professional involved notes on the CDRC how much controlled drug remains and how it will be destroyed—either in the home with a witness, or returning it to a pharmacist who will sign for it, or by asking the family to return it to a pharmacist—and then returns a copy of the CDRC to the PCT. By comparing the CDRC copies in conjunction with the patient's medicines record, it will be possible to detect diversion of surplus stocks.

Two successful pilots have been held in which one of the authors (G Brack) was involved (NHS, 2010a and b). The response of nurses was extremely positive. Although it involves some extra paperwork, nurses liked the fact that for the first time they could tell how much controlled drug should be in the patient's home when they first arrive, and they could prove that they had handed any surplus over for destruction, thus avoiding untoward suspicion. However, the other changes that have been made as a result of the Shipman Inquiry were considered to have improved public safety to such an extent that the extra costs of the CDRC system could not be justified by the small additional benefit that it could bring.

There have also been changes to the validity and duration of prescriptions. Now, a prescription for a controlled drug must be dispensed within 28 days of its date (or another date specified by the prescriber if forward-dated) and it is strongly recommended that no more than 30 days' supply should be made on any one form, though the law allows flexibility on this where there is good reason such as the need to cover an extended holiday.

More recently the Care Quality Commission (2012) published their annual report on the safer management of controlled drugs, which contains several recommendations pertinent to the role of the accountable officer. They also encourage the use of a standard Controlled Drug Requisition form.

In August 2012 the Human Medicines Regulations came into force. They simplify medicines legislation; replacing much of the Medicines Act and other statutory instruments. The regulations also introduce some policy changes to ensure legislation reflects modern medicines management. New European Union (EU) legislation on monitoring the safety of medicines is incorporated into these regulations.

The legal roles of various health professionals

Safe, appropriate, and effective medicines management is not solely the role of the nurse. It is essential that a multidisciplinary approach is taken. This means ensuring that all members of the healthcare team involved in the management of the patient, the patient, and their carers are involved and aware of what is happening. There are many different legal mechanisms for the supply and administration of medicines, which will now be described.

The prescribing, dispensing, supply, and administration of medicines

Each registrant on the Nursing and Midwifery Council's register of nurses is accountable for their actions whether prescribing, dispensing, supplying or administering a medicine/medicinal product and also when delegating to others to do so (NMC, 2010), (HPC, 2008).

Table 1.2 Differences between the prescribing, dispensing, supply, and administration of medicines.

Mechanism for getting the medicine to the patient	Definition	Who can do what?
Prescribing	Written instructions for the dispensing/supply/administration of medicines/medicinal products from a registered professional who is licensed/authorized by their professional body	A medical practitioner (doctor or dentist); a non-medical prescriber (see 'Prescribing and non-medical prescribers' for more information).
Dispensing	Labelling from stock and supplying medicine/medicinal product to a patient, following the instructions of a written prescription (not a patient group direction)	Registered nurses*, pharmacists, and health professionals
Supply	To give a medicine/medicinal products to a patient following the instructions of a written prescription	Registered nurses, pharmacists, and health professionals and students who have been assessed as competent to do so
Administration	The act of giving a medicinal product to a patient under the instructions of a written prescription	Registered nurses, pharmacists, and health professionals and students who have been assessed as competent to do so

* The nurse's ability to dispense is restricted to giving hospital patients medicines to take home on discharge, but increasingly Trusts are arranging that all dispensing should be done within pharmacies. This may mean that they are prepared some distance away and the nurse's role is restricted to checking that the right patient is given the sealed bag that has been delivered from the pharmacy. NMC (2007)

These terms all refer to mechanisms that are regulated by law as ways to ensure that a patient gets their medicine. They are not interchangeable and there are significant legal differences. Definitions of the terms are set out in Table 1.2.

You will see that while these roles are normally performed by different people, it is possible that the same person could undertake more than one. This would potentially remove one of the important safeguards that keep patients safe.

Ordinarily, a doctor (or non-medical prescriber) prescribes a medicine, and a pharmacist dispenses it. This means that a second professional has the opportunity to intervene if the prescription is unclear or unsafe. If a nurse becomes a non-medical prescriber and prescribes a medicine which they themselves will administer to the patient, there is a risk that any mistakes made will not be corrected. For this reason, the NMC *Standards of Proficiency for Nurse and Midwife Prescribers* (2006) p 25 state that:

9.1 You must ensure separation of prescribing and administering activities whenever possible

and

9.2 In the exceptional circumstance, where you are involved in both prescribing and administering a patient/client's controlled drug, a second suitably competent person should be involved in checking the accuracy of the medication provided.

Prescribing and non-medical prescribers

Prescribers fall into two categories, medical prescribers, as in a registered doctor or dentist, and non-medical prescribers. To prescribe a medicine or medicinal product the health professional must be registered with their professional body and must first have undertaken the appropriate training and have been granted by their professional body authorization or a licence to prescribe from the formulary that is linked to their recordable qualification (NMC, 2006). A list of health professionals other than medical practitioners (doctors/dentists) who are able to prescribe as non-medical prescribers and their prescribing rights can be accessed by using the following URL: **http://www.dh.gov.uk/en/Publicationsandstatistics/Publications/PublicationsPolicyAndGuidance/DH_064325**.

Material on non-medical prescribing in Scotland can be found at: **http://www.scotland.gov.uk/Topics/Health/NHS-Scotland/non-medicalprescribing/policy**.

All prescribers are accountable under their professional codes of conduct and ethics for their prescribing decisions, actions, and omissions. Non-medical prescribers are accountable under their respective codes of conduct and ethics to their professional bodies (NMC 2008), (HPC, 2008), (Royal Pharmaceutical Society for Great Britain (RPSGB), 2007). The Nursing and Midwifery Council has produced a set of *Standards for Nurse and Midwife Prescribers* (NMC, 2006), these standards also apply to designated registered health professionals who are prescribers; they can be accessed via the following URL: **http://www.nmc-uk.org/Documents/NMC-Publications/NMC-Standards-proficiency-nurse-and-midwife-prescribers.pdf**.

Non-medical prescribers must be registered with their professional body, and must have successfully undertaken appropriate further training to grant them a recordable qualification which is their licence to prescribe. In addition, to be eligible for the training, they must have been deemed by their employing organization to have an identified service need to prescribe. Depending on their professional registration, their professional role, their competence and scope of practice, and the relevant legislation (see earlier in this chapter), non-medical prescribers can be community practitioner nurse prescribers, independent and supplementary prescribers, or supplementary prescribers alone. Professions other than nurses can become non-medical prescribers, but these will not be discussed further here.

Independent prescribers

As independent prescribers, non-medical prescribers can prescribe any licensed medicine and as a result of changes to the Medicines for Human Use legislation in 2009, nurse independent prescribers can also prescribe unlicensed medicines that are within their formulary, provided that they are clinically competent to do so (NMC, 2010). As well as being clinically competent, the non-medical independent prescriber must be confident to prescribe as they are accountable for having fully assessed the patient and made a diagnosis and for any prescribing decisions and actions regardless of whether they write a prescription or not. For example, they are accountable for the advice they give to the patient regarding how and when to take their medication, to start or stop medication, and also for whether they tell the patient to buy their medicines from a pharmacy. Non-medical independent prescribing is well used by advanced health practitioners who are running their own clinics where they carry a responsibility for assessing patients and making a diagnosis. When prescribing unlicensed drugs, non-medical independent prescribers must have a strong rationale for doing so, having fully assessed the patient and made a diagnosis and, as with any drug that they prescribe, the support of their employing organization.

Supplementary prescribing

Supplementary prescribing is defined by the Department of Health ((DH), 2006) as a voluntary partnership between the patient, a non-medical prescriber and an independent prescriber who has to be a medical practitioner (doctor or a dentist). For legislation in Northern Ireland see the Department of Health, Social Services, and Public Safety website: **http://www.dhsspsni.gov.uk/non-medical-prescribing**.

The medical practitioner independent prescriber and the supplementary prescriber are responsible for agreeing a clinical management plan (CMP) which must be set up with the knowledge of the patient/carer in advance of the patient's care.

Supplementary prescribing is a useful tool for advanced health practitioners caring for patients with long term conditions where the supplementary prescriber is clinically competent and competent to prescribe but would value the ongoing supervision of the independent prescriber to support prescribing confidence.

In the case of supplementary prescribing, the medical practitioner who is the independent prescriber is responsible for the overall care of the patient and for having made the initial diagnosis. The diagnosis must be agreed by the supplementary prescriber or else they will not be able to prescribe. Once the CMP has been agreed and is in place, the supplementary prescriber can prescribe any drug or range/category of drugs indicated on the plan and by any route or within any dose range that has been written on the plan. The supplementary prescriber is accountable for having agreed the plan and for any prescribing decisions they make whilst working under the plan. If the supplementary prescriber identifies a need to prescribe something that is not on the plan they must either:

- refer to the medical practitioner independent prescriber who will prescribe for the patient or
- they must negotiate a new plan with the medical practitioner independent prescriber or
- if they are also a non-medical independent prescriber, they can prescribe for the patient, providing they are clinically competent and confident to do so.

By range or category of drugs, we mean that the CMP does not have to name all the drugs individually, provided it is made clear which medicines are included. For example, the CMP could specify that the supplementary prescriber can prescribe 'an emollient cream', which would allow them to select the one they preferred, or to change the selection at intervals without needing a new plan. It could also refer to a list in a formulary, or the drugs in a particular chapter of the *British National Formulary*. The important point is that there must be no doubt as to whether a particular medicine is permitted or not. Remember that a supplementary prescriber has no legal authority to prescribe anything that is not permitted by the CMP.

More information about CMPs can be accessed on the following URLs: **http://www.dh.gov.uk/en/ Healthcare/Medicinespharmacyandindustry/ Prescriptions/TheNon-MedicalPrescribingPro- gramme/Supplementaryprescribing/DH_4123030**

and **http://www.rosalieboyce.com.au/Alison-Hogg-papers/DH_clinical_management_plans.pdf**.

A list of health professionals who are able to prescribe as non-medical prescribers and their prescribing rights can be accessed by clicking on the following link: **http://www.dh.gov.uk/en/Publica- tionsandstatistics/Publications/PublicationsPoli- cyAndGuidance/DH_064325**.

Who can administer drugs?

Non-medical prescribers must always have assessed the patient themselves before making a prescribing decision and acting as a prescriber. The NMC (2006) *Standards of Proficiency for Nurse and Midwife Prescribers* state that as a nurse or midwife prescriber:

> **You may delegate the administration of a medication that you have prescribed. You remain accountable for your actions and you must be sure the person to whom you have delegated is competent and has received sufficient training to administer the prescribed medication. (Practice standard 14.1 p 26.)**

The HPC *Standards of Conduct Performance and Ethics* (2008) state that as a registrant:

> **You are responsible for the appropriateness of your decision to delegate a task (p 8).**

This links to the NMC (2010) Standards for Medicines Management standard 17, p 40 that adds:

> **A registrant is responsible for the delegation of any aspects of the administration of medicinal products and they are accountable to ensure that the patient or carer/care assistant is competent to carry out the task.**

Therefore student nurses and midwives and health professional students who are studying for professional registration, as long as they have been assessed by a registered professional as being competent to do so, can administer medicines that have been prescribed (with the exception of medicines/drugs that are to be supplied or administered as part of a patient group direction, see section on PGDs).

Prescriptions

Examples of dummy prescription forms used by non-medical prescribers in primary care in the different regions of the UK can be seen in Figures 1.1, 1.2, and 1.3. Nurses may also use green prescriptions as used by general practitioners, but they must only use their own forms.

A number of different prescription forms are used within the NHS. These differ according to the type of prescriber and the country in which they are issued. You can see examples of current and past prescription forms for England at **http://www.nhsbsa.nhs. uk/PrescriptionServices/Documents/Prescription-Services/Current_and_Out_of_Date_Rx_Form_Published_0709.pdf**.

Welsh prescription forms are similar, but bilingual. Scottish forms and those used in Northern Irish forms contain the same information in a slightly different layout.

Prescriptions used in hospitals do not follow a single format. It is important that you familiarize yourself with the forms used in your hospital so that you know where to find all the information you will need. Similarly, with the exception of prescriptions for controlled drugs, prescriptions in private practice do not have a standard format. They must contain the same details as an NHS prescription, plus an indication of the qualifications of the prescriber so that the dispensing pharmacist can check that they have authority to prescribe.

Patient group directions and patient specific directions

What are patient group directions?

A patient group direction (PGD) is the legal term for a written instruction from an authorizing doctor who is acting as an independent prescriber and who is working at a directorate level within their healthcare organization. The direction is designed to enable certain registered health professionals (whose profession has been identified as part of the PGD) to supply or administer drugs and medication in line with the strict instructions set out within the PGD. The patient may or may not be identified by name before they come for their treatment (DH, 2006). The key is that they can be identified by some shared characteristic—for example, they are likely to need anti-tetanus treatment because they have received a penetrating injury or emergency hormonal contraception because they have a risk of pregnancy following unprotected sex; they form part of an identifiable patient group.

In the case of a PGD a prescription does not need to be written for each individual administration of the drug or medicine. PGDs are written usually for the one off or short term supply or administration of medicines in a specific clinical situation; for example, for the administration of trimethoprim for a urinary infection in a minor illness walk-in clinic. If the condition persists the patient should be advised to consult with their doctor or another health professional who is a prescriber.

The registered health professional has an accountability to work under the specific instructions that have been set down in the PGD. The clinical boundaries of the PGD are clearly defined; the condition is named, the drug and dose range are named, and the length of time for administration and number of doses that can be administered are clearly defined. Failure on the part of a registered health professional to comply with the specific written instructions contained within a PGD could result in prosecution under the Medicines Act 1968, because that would be a supply of a prescription only medicine without proper authority. Registered health professionals who supply or administer drugs and medicines under a PGD must be clinically competent and must work under their code of conduct (NMC, 2008). Registered health professionals have to be assessed by their manager in their clinical setting as being competent to supply or administer the medicines under the PGD (NMC, 2010). The registered professional must sign the PGD to indicate that they have read and understand the directions and they are clinically competent to supply or administer the drug. An appropriate person—usually the registrant's clinical

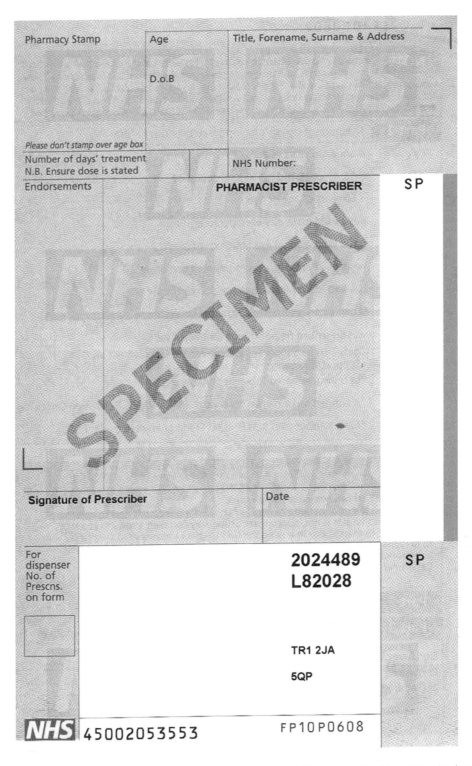

Figure 1.1 An example of a prescription. Nurses may also use green prescriptions as used by GPs, but must only use their own forms.

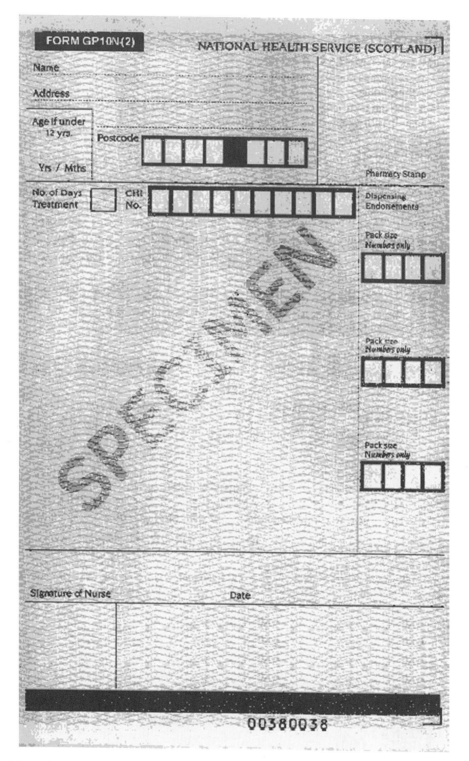

Figure 1.2 A Scottish nurse prescriber's form.

Courtesy of NHS Scotland, © Crown Copyright.

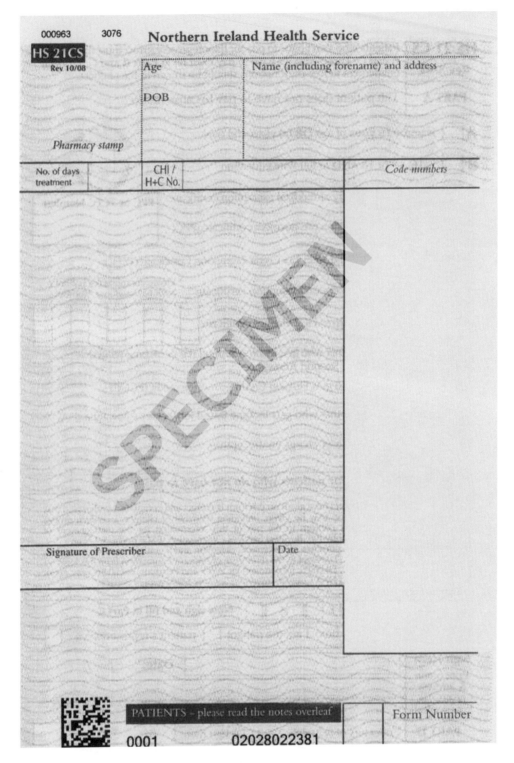

Figure 1.3 A nurse prescribing form from Northern Ireland.

line manager—must sign that they have assessed the registrant as being competent to supply or administer under the PGD and that they are satisfied that the registrant has understood the directions. PGDs are for the supply or administration of licensed drugs only, but can be used for off-licence use of licensed drugs (NHS, 2009). Note also that a PGD is not needed when the medicine is not a prescription only medicine, because a PGD is defined in law as 'a written direction for the supply and administration of a description or class of prescription only medicines . . .' (POM amendment order SI 2000/1917, s. 2(a)).

The Department of Health has listed the registered professionals who are able to supply or administer under PGDs as being:

- Nurses
- Midwives
- Optometrists
- Pharmacists
- Chiropodists/podiatrists
- Radiographers
- Physiotherapists
- Paramedics
- Dieticians
- Occupational therapists
- Speech and language therapists
- Orthotists (DH, 2006).

PGDs are of most use in areas where the patient has not already been identified and in areas such as minor injury and minor illness walk-in clinics or in out-of-hours clinics where a prescriber is not immediately accessible, for example in:

- Minor injury (pain control)
- Minor Illness (one off treatment of infection with antibiotics prior to the patient seeing a prescriber)
- Emergency situations (emergency paramedicine)
- Family planning clinics (emergency hormonal contraception)
- Vaccination clinics

More registered health professionals are now qualifying as prescribers, and PGDs are in the process of being phased out by some health care organizations.

Students and patient group directions

Health professional and nursing students are not permitted under law to supply or administer drugs/medicines under the instructions of a PGD even if they are directly supervised by their mentor. The Nursing and Midwifery Council (2009a) have issued a circular regarding the position of students in relation to PGDs. This circular is to be read and acted on in conjunction with the professional code of conduct (NMC, 2008), the Essential Skills Cluster (NMC, 2007) and the Standards for Medicines Management (NMC, 2010). This circular also applies to students who are studying for other health professional qualifications and these students would need to take into account their own professional codes. This is because only registered health professionals whose profession has been named on the written PGD are legally allowed to supply or administer the drug/medication that is named on the PGD (DH, 2006).

The registrant is accountable to the law, their employer, the prescriber, and to their professional body and responsible for the supply or administration of the medicine/drug. The registered professional cannot therefore delegate a student to supply or administer a drug under their instructions even if they directly supervise the student. You can use Exercise 1.2 to help you examine some PGDs.

Box 1.2

Only registered health professionals whose profession has been named on a written PGD are legally allowed to supply or administer the drug/medication that is named on the PGD.

Patient specific directions (what are they and who can do what?)

A patient specific direction (PSD) is a written instruction from a prescriber for a drug/medicine to be

Exercise 1.2

When in clinical placement:

- Try to locate the PGDs that apply to your clinical area and make a list of them.
- Are these stored electronically or are there paper versions?
- What conditions are they for?
- What are the drugs that can be supplied or administered?
- Who are the registered professionals that can legally supply or administer drugs under the PGD?
- Who is individually signed up to supply/administer under the PGD?
- What are the boundaries of the PGD?
- What is the expiry date on the PGD?

supplied or administered to a named patient. The PSD must include:

- The name of the patient
- The name of the drug
- The drug dosage
- The formulation of the drug/medication (how it is made up) for example tablet or solution
- The frequency of administration
- The duration for which the drug/medication is to be given for
- The total overall dose of the drug/medication to be supplied.

The PSD must be written by the prescriber and there must be a contemporaneous recording of this within the patient's medical record. PSDs can take the form of a handwritten or electronic instruction. An example can be found in Box 1.3.

PSDs are used when the patient or patients are known in advance of the prescription being acted upon; for example, where there is a clinic list for the administration of a set vaccination where both the names of the patients are listed and the drugs to be administered, their frequency, and their dosages are listed. The doctor authorizing the vaccination need only sign once for the whole patient list.

Box 1.3 Example of a PSD

Mr X.
DOB: 20.10.60
Address: 3 The Lane, Big Town. BT3 9JR
10 mg of exirtionmycin (made up drug name). To be given four times a day at six hourly intervals.
Give one tablet every six hours for five days. Supply 20 tablets.(Signature of the prescriber).

The registered professional who is supplying or administering under a PSD is accountable for their actions. The registered health professional who is delegated the task of supplying or administering a drug/medication as a result of a PSD is not directly named, therefore a health care worker or student can supply or administer under a PSD providing that they are under the direct supervision of a registered professional who is acting as their mentor and who carries the accountability for having delegated the task.

A PSD is a written instruction and verbal instructions are not acceptable. Table 1.3 illustrates the differences between a PGD and a PSD. An NHS prescription form is one form of PSD.

To check your understanding, you may wish to tackle a short quiz on PGDs. The answers may be found at the end of this chapter.

Quiz

1 What does the abbreviation PGD stand for?

a) Patient group prescription?

b) Patient group directive?

c) Prescribing group direction?

d) Patient group direction?

2 A PGD can be defined as:

a) An authorized direction for the dispensing of a medicinal product?

b) An authorized direction for the supply or administration of a medicinal product?

Table 1.3 The differences between a patient group direction (PGD) and a patient specific direction (PSD).

Indication	Patient group direction	Patient specific direction	Space for you to write your own comments
For a named clinical condition	√	√	
Patients must be known in advance of the prescription being supplied or administered		√	
Must be signed by a prescriber	√	√	
The supply or administration can be delegated by the prescriber	√	√	
The supply or administration can be delegated by a registered professional who is competent to supply or administer the drug		√	
The person who is supplying or administering the drug must be competent to do so	√	√	
The person who is designated to supply or administer the drug must be a named and registered health professional	√		

c) An authorized direction for giving the patient a prescription?

d) A protocol for the management of a clinical condition?

3 Who can work under a PGD?

a) Student nurses and health professionals?

b) Patients?

c) Carers?

d) Designated registered health professionals?

4 What does the term PSD stand for?

a) Patient standing prescription?

b) Person specific direction?

c) Patient specific direction?

d) Prescriber specific direction?

5 A registered health professional who is authorized to supply or administer a drug/medicine under PSD:

a) Must be clinically competent to do so?

b) Can delegate this task to a student who is under their direct supervision?

c) Must refuse to delegate this task to any other person

d) Is not directly accountable for their actions.

Patients and their legal rights

This section will outline the various legal rights that patients have in respect of medicines. These are no different to those for other forms of treatment.

Patient consent

The underlying principle of consent is very simple and was thus described by the American judge Benjamin Cardozo:

> **Every human being of adult years and sound mind has a right to determine what shall be done with his own body; and a surgeon who performs an operation without his patient's consent commits an assault for which he is liable in damages.**
> *Schloendorff v Society of New York Hospital* (1914).

It is not necessary to hurt someone to commit an assault. Indeed, it is not even necessary to make contact. An assault can be committed if a person reasonably thinks that they are about to be touched without their consent. Once the person is touched, the offence of battery may be committed.

It is necessary to have the patient's consent to anything that we do to them to protect us against an allegation of assault. Nurses are very used to seeing patients being asked to sign consent forms before surgery, but the same requirement exists for the giving of medicine.

A patient can signal consent without signing a form. If you are running a vaccination clinic, and your patient rolls up their sleeve and offers you their arm, that is implied consent. You are entitled to believe that their actions show that they are consenting to the treatment that you are offering.

Usually when nurses are conducting a medicine round, the patient already knows the medicines that will be offered because the prescriber should have obtained their consent to being treated in this way. However, if an adult patient of sound mind refuses their medication, their wish must be respected. They have withdrawn their consent, and it would be improper, and probably unlawful, to force them to have a treatment that they have refused. It does not matter that they will suffer harm without it, provided that they understood the consequences of refusing the medication.

To be valid, the consent must be informed. Occasionally the term 'informed consent' is used, but if consent was not informed, it cannot be a valid consent. A patient who is asked to consent to treatment must be given all the relevant information that they need to make an informed decision, and their questions must be answered fully and honestly. If you cannot answer a question, you perform your duty by finding someone who can answer it.

There have been rare examples of health professionals being allowed to withhold information from patients on the grounds that it may cause them unreasonable distress, but courts are increasingly unlikely to take this view. See, for example, guidance on consent from the GMC, available at: **http://www.gmc-uk.org/guidance/ethical_guidance/**
consent_guidance_reasons_for_not_sharing_information.asp.

Exercise 1.3

If you were a patient, what would you want to know before agreeing to a treatment?

You might include:

- What benefit will this treatment give me?
- What adverse effects might I suffer, and how likely are they?
- How might this treatment interact with other treatments I might be having?
- Will this treatment affect my life? For example, will it make me sleepy, or unable to work?
- Are there features of the treatment that may not be obvious to a layperson that a healthcare professional would take for granted? For example, will I have to come back to hospital for future doses, or can I have them at home?
- Are there any other factors of the proposed treatment that might affect my decision?

While Justice Cardozo's statement spoke of adults, it is now settled law in the United Kingdom that people under 18 can also give consent. Under the Family Law Reform Act (1969), section 8(1), a person over 16 is treated as an adult for the purposes of giving consent to medical treatment. If this were not so, a woman who married perfectly legally at 16 would have to ask her parent or guardian to consent to the provision of a contraceptive. Since the case of *Gillick v West Norfolk and Wisbech Area Health Authority* (1985) it has been clear that a minor under 16 can also give consent if he or she understands what is involved. Lord Scarman expressed it thus:

> **As a matter of Law the parental right to determine whether or not their minor child below the age of sixteen will have medical treatment terminates if and when the child achieves sufficient understanding and intelligence to understand fully what is proposed.**
>
> (Gillick, 1985)

When a child is not mature enough to give consent, an adult with appropriate authority can do so for them. This will usually be the parent or guardian. It is not necessary to ask both parents—consent is only needed from one person entitled to give it.

There is no such general rule for adults who lack capacity (are unable to make decisions for themselves). Courts have held that the duty of healthcare professionals in those circumstances is to act in the patient's best interests, and this principle is now enshrined in legislation (see next paragraph). This is not restricted to best medical interests. It is this provision that allows us to give emergency treatment in cases of necessity without waiting for consent—think how difficult it would be to resuscitate a patient whose heart had stopped if we had to find a relative to give consent before we started.

Although not legally necessary, it is common to consult the patient's family in such cases. This sometimes results in the family saying that they believe they know what their relative would have wanted. This is called substituted judgement and can be fraught with difficulty because it is hard to be sure that their judgement is right. It is not unknown for a mother's children to disagree strongly about 'what mother would have wanted'. For this reason the law in the UK favours the best interest test over the substituted judgement test (Foster, 2011).

However, there are two circumstances in which we can be sure of the patient's wishes. Sometimes a person may have prepared an advance decision (sometimes known as a 'living will') in which they will say that if a particular set of circumstances comes about and they are no longer able to make a decision for themselves, they want a particular course of action to be followed. They cannot insist upon a treatment being given, but they can say that they would accept or refuse it if offered. For example, a person could say that if they are attached to a life support system with no prospect of improvement in their condition, they want it switched off.

Alternatively, the patient can appoint someone as a proxy to make decisions on their behalf. Under the Mental Capacity Act (2005) a person can create a Lasting Power of Attorney (LPA) appointing a named person to make decisions for them about a range of subjects including their health. This applies to England and Wales. In Scotland, the Adults with Incapacity (Scotland) Act (2000b) contains similar provisions, but there the term 'Welfare Power of Attorney' is used instead. Northern Ireland does not yet have the same provision.

The Scottish legislation can be read at **http://www.legislation.gov.uk/asp/2000/4/contents**.

There is a simple guide to the law in England and Wales at **http://www.dca.gov.uk/menincap/mca-act-easyread.pdf**.

A more detailed discussion is given by Bartlett (2005).

There are criteria for deciding whether someone has capacity to make their own decisions. These lie outside the scope of this book—here we need only note that we cannot say someone lacks capacity just because they make a surprising decision or one that may harm them.

In certain circumstances a person may be assessed or treated without their consent under The Mental Health Act (1983), particularly if they may be a danger to others.

Access to medicines

Patients do not have the right to demand any particular treatment. However, if a treatment is available in a particular place, patients should have equal access to it. This is required by the NHS Constitution (Department of Health, 2012) which does not allow public bodies to discriminate when offering treatment. Courts have consistently agreed that it is not their place to tell the NHS how to use its resources, but they have been prepared to review decisions that have been made to check that the procedures have been fair and open.

Where the National Institute for Health and Clinical Excellence (NICE) has decided that a treatment should be offered within the NHS, Trusts must make it available. For NICE technology appraisals of such treatments, there is a time limit of three months for introducing them. Longer periods will be needed to implement NICE clinical guidelines, but Trusts that take unreasonable time to make these changes will be criticized by their monitoring organizations.

NICE can be accessed by clicking on **http://www. nice.org.uk/**.

Disability Discrimination Act (1995) and the Equality Act (2010)

Under this legislation we are required to make reasonable adjustments to allow disabled people to use our services. In the case of medicines, this is normally quite straightforward. For example, the pharmacy may have to produce large print labels for poorly-sighted patients, or nurses may have to help patients to open bottles if they cannot do so themselves. Most of these adjustments will be made by the pharmacy, but in some cases the pharmacist will not know that the patient is disabled or the degree of their disability unless someone tells them. If pre-registration nurses become aware that someone cannot use their medication properly because they are disabled, they should report the matter to their supervisor.

Vicarious liability

Vicarious liability is sometimes mentioned in relation to legal duties. Unfortunately, sometimes this important legal principle is not properly understood. Vicarious liability is based on the principle that a servant's acts are dictated by his master, so liability for them should rest with the master. In modern terms, the employer is liable for the acts of employees that form part of their duties (Stevens, 2007). This is useful for anyone harmed, who can sue the employing Trust rather than the individual nurse, because the Trust will normally have more money to pay any damages awarded.

However, there are two important limitations to the protection that vicarious liability can offer nurses. First, it extends to the legitimate duties of a nurse. If a nurse does something outside those duties, then a court would have to decide if that was so unconnected with their normal duties that the nurse was actually acting on their own. For example, if a nurse removed sutures despite not being trained, they might be covered by vicarious liability because nurses may remove sutures, even though they should not; but if a nurse removed a patient's appendix they would not be covered, because that is not a nurse's role.

Second, vicarious liability does not apply to criminal acts. There is a fuller discussion of the scope of vicarious liability in Stevens (2007).

What nurses need to know about medicines management

As you can see from the earlier sections, health professionals and patients have various legal responsibilities for medicines management. This extends to setting a standard of minimum knowledge regarding medicines management that health professionals including newly registered nurses should demonstrate they have. In this section we will examine the skills that the NMC has decided that a nurse should have in order to be entered on their registers.

NMC essential skills clusters related to medicines management

The NMC define 'medicines management' as 'The clinical cost effective and safe use of medicines to ensure patients get maximum benefit from the medicines they need while at the same time minimizing potential harm'. (NMC, 2010, p4) and, within the essential skills clusters (ESCs) (NMC, 2007) for pre-registration nursing programmes, set out the requirements for newly registered nurses to achieve this. Nursing programmes need to ensure that students achieve the necessary skills for entry to the particular branch and to the register (see Table 1.4).

In order to gain these skills pre-registration nursing students need to increase their knowledge and experience through a range of learning opportunities in clinical practice and within their programme. Chapters in this book which will help increase your understanding of the principles of medicines management are identified in Table 1.4.

Reflection point

Consider your experiences to date and identify your main learning needs.
Note the chapters within this book that can help you achieve the necessary learning.

Table 1.4 Medicines management essential skills cluster.

Patients/clients can trust a newly registered nurse to:	For further information on this topic see Chapter:
Correctly and safely undertake medicines calculations	7
Work within the legal and ethical framework that underpins safe and effective medicines management	1, 2, 5, and 6
Work as part of a team to offer a range of treatment options of which medicines may form a part	1, 2, 6, and 8
Ensure safe and effective practice through comprehensive knowledge of medicines, their actions, risks, and benefits	3, 4, and 5
Order, receive, store, and dispose of medicines safely in any setting (including controlled drugs)	6
Administer medicines safely and in a timely manner, including controlled drugs	1, 2, 3, and 5
Keep and maintain accurate records within a multi-disciplinary framework and as part of a team	1, 6
Work in partnership with patients/clients and carers in relation to concordance and managing their medicines	8
Use and evaluate up-to-date information on medicines management and work within national and local policies	1, 2, and 5
Demonstrate understanding and knowledge to supply and administer via a patient group direction (PGD)	1

Basic principle of medicines management: giving the right medicine to the right person in the right dose at the right time

The main aim of medicines management is to achieve the desired therapeutic effect for the patient. In order to do this you need to

- give the correct medicine,
- at the correct dose,
- to the correct person,
- in the correct formulation,
- by the correct route, and
- at the correct time intervals.

As student nurses you will no doubt have these phrases memorized, but stop for a moment to reflect on practice.

Reflection point

Think of examples when you know this has not been achieved. What were the reasons?

The reasons for errors will be explored further in Chapter 2.

It is vital that you administer medicines to achieve the desired therapeutic effect 100% of the time, recognising that it is not a mechanised task and must involve an understanding of the written prescription (NMC, 2010). An understanding of the underlying principles of pharmacology and patient safety are essential.

Medicine administration is the final step in a multidisciplinary process in which professionals should work together to ensure that the various stages are properly integrated so that the correct medicine is safely administered to the patient. It is your responsibility to work with colleagues to maintain the safety of those in your care (NMC, 2008). An important aspect of working with others is recording the care you have delivered so others have access to this information.

Clear and accurate records of all medicines administered must be made immediately. Documentation should also include when a medicine has not been administered and the reason for this identified. Registrants who delegate the task of administration of medicines remain responsible, not only for the task but also for documentation. Similarly, when supervising a student nurse participating in medicines management, a registrant is responsible for clearly countersigning the signature of the student.

NMC standards for medicines administration

For registrants the NMC make very clear your responsibilities for practice in the *Standards for Medicines Management* (NMC, 2010). Use the following link to access this document: **http://www.nmc-uk.org/Documents/NMC-Publications/NMC-Standards-for-medicines-management.pdf**.

The first priority prior to administering any medicine is to check the 'direction to supply or administer' the medication. Written instructions for the administration of medicines or medicinal products must be from a registered professional who is licensed/authorized by their professional body. As has already been discussed earlier in this chapter, this written instruction can be provided in several ways. Those working within a secondary care setting will be familiar with patient medicine administration charts, which provide a direction to administer medication. It must be signed by a registered prescriber but it must be remembered that it is the registrant who is accountable for the administration of the prescribed medicine.

Standard 1 of the NMC *Standards for Medicines Management* (2010) clearly states that registrants must only administer medicines if one of the following written directions is in place:

- Patient specific direction (PSD)
- Patient medicines administration chart or medicines administration record

- Patient group direction (PGD)
- Medicines act exemption (where they apply to nurses)
- Standing order
- Homely remedy protocol
- Prescription forms

NMC (2010, p 13)

A homely remedy protocol is used in care homes. It lists medicines such as a resident might have in their own home and authorizes use of those medicines without a specific direction from a doctor for a short period of time. Medicines included are likely to be a mild laxative, an indigestion mixture, paracetamol tablets, an anti-diarrhoea preparation, and a simple cough mixture.

You will find that NHS Trust policies frequently highlight that in the interests of patient safety and clinical governance, medicines must NOT be administered against verbal prescriptions.

Exercise 1.4

Check your local policy regarding the administration of medicines.

Registrants should only administer medicines in line with the basic principles of medicines management, identified earlier in this chapter. You must be certain of the identity of the patient to whom the medicine is to be administered, as well as having considered the dosage, weight of patient where appropriate, method of administration, route, and timing.

However, in acknowledgement that administration of medicines is a more complex process, the following factors are implicit:

- Check that the patient is not allergic to the medicine before administering it.
- Know the therapeutic uses of the medicine to be administered, its normal dosage, side effects, precautions, and contraindications

- Check that the prescription and the label on the medicine are clear and unambiguous
- Check expiry date on the medicine.

It is also the responsibility of the registrant to assess the patient's condition prior to administration to ensure appropriateness of administration. For example, digoxin is not usually to be given if the patient's pulse rate is below 60 beats per minute. If assessment indicates that the medicine is no longer appropriate or a contraindication is noted then the person who has prescribed the medicine must be contacted quickly. Similarly, they must be contacted if the patient develops a reaction.

Summary

In this chapter these points have been addressed:

- The key legislation relating to medicines including the Medicines Act and the Misuse of Drugs Act
- What is meant by 'controlled drugs' and the regulations relating to their storage and use
- What is meant by 'nurse prescriber'
- When a student nurse can administer drugs and how this should be undertaken
- The meanings of and differences between patient group directions (PGDs) and patient specific directions (PSDs).
- The meaning of accountability and responsibility and how these relate to the administration and supply of medicines

References

Bartlett P (2005), *Blackstone's Guide to the Mental Capacity Act 2005*. Oxford: Oxford University Press.

BNF see Joint Formulary Committee.

Bosely S (2010), Fifty Years on, an apology to thalidomide scandal survivors. Available at: http://www.guardian.co.uk/society/2010/jan/14/thalidomide-apology-government (accessed 28 June 2012).

Brown M (2009), Will the sacking of drugs expert Professor David Nutt deter other scientists from advising government? http://blogs.telegraph.co.uk/news/andrewmcfbrown/100015335/will-the-sacking-of-professor-david-nutt-deter-other-scientists-from-advising-government/ (accessed 28 June 2012).

Department of Health (2006), *Medicines Matters: A guide to the mechanisms for the prescribing, supply and administration of medicines*. Available at http://www.dh.gov.uk/en/Publicationsandstatistics/Publications/PublicationsPolicyAndGuidance/DH_064325 (accessed 15 February 2012).

Department of Health (2012), *The NHS Constitution*. Available at http://www.dh.gov.uk/en/Publicationsandstatistics/Publications/PublicationsPolicyAndGuidance/DH_132961 (accessed 1 May 2012).

Department of Health, Social Services and Public Safety (Northern Ireland) at: http://www.dhsspsni.gov.uk/non-medical-prescribing (accessed 21 September 2012).

European Council, Directive 2004/27/EC of the European Parliament and of the Council of 31 March 2004 amending Directive 2001/83/EC on the Community code relating to medicinal products for human use. Available at http://ec.europa.eu/health/files/eudralex/vol-1/dir_2004_27/dir_2004_27_en.pdf (accessed 9 July 2012).

Foster C (2011), *Human Dignity in Bioethics and Law*. Oxford: Oxford University Press.

Gillick v West Norfolk and Wisbech Area Health Authority [1985] 3 All ER 402 (HL) p 423.

Health Professions Council (2008), *Standards of Conduct, Performance and Ethics*. London: HPC.

HMSO (1919), *The Treaty of Peace between the Allied and Associated Powers and Germany*, London.

Joint Formulary Committee (2012). *British National Formulary* (64th ed). London: BMJ Group and Pharmaceutical Press.

League of Nations Treaty Series (1922), No. 222. *International Opium Convention*. Signed at The Hague. January 23, 1912. Available at http://www.worldlii.org/int/other/LNTSer/1922/29.html (accessed 28 June 2012).

NHS (2009), *Patient Group Directions* Liverpool: National Prescribing Centre.

NHS (2010a), *Review of the Implementation of the Controlled Drugs Record Card (Phase 1)* Liverpool: National Prescribing Centre.

NHS (2010b), *Recommendations in Response to the CDRC Implementation Review*. Liverpool: National Prescribing Centre.

Nursing and Midwifery Council (2006), *Standards of Proficiency for Nurse and Midwife Prescribers*. London: NMC.

Nursing and Midwifery Council (2007), *Essential Skills Clusters (ESC) for Pre-registration Nursing Programmes*. NMC Circular 07/2007. London: NMC.

Nursing and Midwifery Council (2008), *The Code. Standards of Conduct, Performance and Ethics for Nurses and Midwives*. London: NMC.

Nursing and Midwifery Council (2009a), *Supply and/or Administration of Medicine by Student Nurses and Student Midwives in Relation to Patient Group Directions (PGDs)*. NMC Circular 05/2009. London: NMC.

Nursing and Midwifery Council (2009b), *Guidance on Professional Conduct for Nursing and Midwifery Students: your Guide to Practice*. London; NMC.

Nursing and Midwifery Council (2010), *Standards for Medicines Management*. London: NMC.

Pendergrast M (2000), *For God, Country and Coca-Cola: The Definitive History of the Great American Soft Drink and the Company That Makes It*. Basic Books: New York.

Royal Pharmaceutical Society for Great Britain (2007), *Code of Ethics for Pharmacists and Pharmacy Technicians*. London: RPSGB.

Schloendorff v Society of New York Hospital (1914), 211 NY 125, 105 NE 92. Available at: http://sc.judiciary.gov.ph/jurisprudence/2011/june2011/165279_carpio.html (accessed 18 November 2012).

Scottish Government (2006), Information on non-medical prescribing available on: http://www.scotland.gov.uk/Topics/Health/NHS-Scotland/non-medicalprescribing/policy (accessed 18 November 2012).

Smith J (2004), *Shipman Inquiry 5th Report: Safeguarding Patients: Lessons from the Past–Proposals for the Future*, Cm 6394, paragraphs 18.166–18.175. HMSO: London.

Stevens R (2007), *Torts and Rights*. Oxford: Oxford University Press.

Streatfeild D (2003), *Cocaine: An Unauthorized Biography*, London: Macmillan. p. 80.

UK legislation referred to in the text

All UK legislation was published in London by The Stationery Office, previously known as His/Her Majesty's Stationery Office.

Adults with Incapacity (Scotland) Act (2000b): http://www.legislation.gov.uk/asp/2000/4/contents (accessed 18 November 2012).

The Dangerous Drugs Act (1920), 10 and 11 Geo. V, c. 46.

The Dangerous Drugs Act (1967), c. 82.

The Defence of the Realm Act (1914), 4 and 5 Geo. V, c.29.

The Disability Discrimination Act (1995), c. 50.

The Equality Act (2010), c. 15.

The Family Law Reform Act (1969), c. 46.

The Medicines Act (1968), c. 67.

The Medicines for Human Use (Miscellaneous Amendments) (no.2) Regulations. SI 2009/3063. Available at: http://www.nmc-uk.org/Documents/Circulars/2010circulars/NMCcircular04_2010.pdf (accessed 18 November 2012).

The Mental Capacity Act (2005), c. 9.

The Mental Health Act (1983), c. 20.

The Misuse of Drugs Act (1971), c. 38.

The Prescription Only Medicines (Human Use) Amendment Order (2000) SI 2000/1917.

Quiz answers

1 d,   **2** b,   **3** d,   **4** c,   **5** b.

2 Patient Safety and Error Reduction

CHAPTER CONTENTS

- How can we reduce the incidence of harm from medication?
- The importance of near misses
- Never events
- What actions most commonly lead to mistakes?
- Reason's Swiss cheese model of errors
- Active failures and latent conditions

- The system approach in action
- Using guidelines and protocols to reduce risks
- Learning from our mistakes
- Serious untoward incident policies
- The national reporting and learning system (NRLS) and the yellow card system
- Personal accountability
- Summary

LEARNING OUTCOMES

By the end of this chapter you should understand:

- The role of the National Patient Safety Agency and how it uses the National Reporting and Learning System
- The burden that medication errors place on the NHS
- Where those errors arise
- Reason's Swiss Cheese model of errors
- How we follow up incidents to learn from them
- How we can use guidelines and protocols to reduce errors
- Significant event analysis
- Why personal accountability is important
- The yellow card system.

Most healthcare professionals take up their career because they want to make people better. It is rare—but not unknown—to find nurses deliberately harming patients. It is not always possible to cure a patient's condition, and readers may be surprised to hear the view of Lord Justice Stuart-Smith that our 'only duty as a matter of law is not to make the victim's condition worse' (*Capital and Counties plc v Hampshire CC* (1997) 2 All ER 865 at 883).

Despite our best intentions, healthcare professionals do sometimes make the patient's condition worse. There are too many instances of harm caused to patients. Not only does the patient suffer harm, staff will be upset (some may even give up their careers) and large compensation claims may be made which deplete NHS resources. According to the NHS Litigation Authority, in 2010–11 it received 8655 claims of clinical negligence and 4346 claims of non-clinical negligence against NHS bodies, and paid £863 million in connection with clinical negligence claims (NHSLA Annual Report and Accounts, 2011). To put that into perspective, NHS Warwickshire had a budget of £827m for that year, so this amount would fund a medium-sized PCT.

For all these reasons, therefore, our first concern must be to do no harm to our patient. If we can improve their condition, so much the better, but at the very least we must leave them no worse off for having put themselves in our care.

Patient safety must be everyone's concern. It is monitored by the NHS Commissioning Board Special Health Authority. Until June 2012 there was a separate agency, the National Patient Safety Agency (NPSA), which produced a report in 2009 entitled *Safety in doses: improving the use of medicines in the NHS*. There were 811746 reports to the NPSA in 2007, of which 86085 were related to medication. The figures for July 2010–June 2011 show an increase to 1.27 million incidents, of which 133727 were related to medication. Data compiled from: **http://www.nrls.npsa.nhs.uk/EasySiteWeb/getresource.axd?AssetID=133437&type=full&servicetype=Attachment**.

That makes medication incidents the second largest category after patient accidents. It may be that this increase is the result of better reporting, but it is still a worrying number. The National Health Service Commissioning Board Special Health Authority maintains responsibility for the National Reporting and Learning System which is used to identify the root cause of patient safety issues. For further information please visit the following web site: **www.nrls.npsa.nhs.uk**.

Incidents are reported through the National Reporting and Learning System (NRLS), a computerized database that collects as much information as possible on each incident and looks for patterns that might help us avoid errors. Fortunately, 96% of the mistakes produced either no harm or negligible harm to patients. All healthcare professionals have a duty to report incidents to NRLS, though in many cases we meet our duty by passing information to a governance manager who undertakes this on behalf of the organization. It is informative to look at the sources of the reports (Table 2.1).

It may be that the patients in hospitals are in poorer health and therefore need more medication. The more medication a person takes, the more chance there is

Table 2.1 Sources of medication incidents reported to NRLS in 2010–2011.

Service	Number of incidents	Percentage
Acute hospitals	96779	73
Community nursing	14545	11
Mental health services	14298	11
Community pharmacy	4329	3
Learning disability	1770	1
General practice	1163	1
Ambulance services	181	0
Community dentistry	34	0
Total	133099	100

NRLS, The national reporting and learning system.

Reflection point

Why do you think so many medication incidents are reported from hospitals?

that something will go wrong. We will examine polypharmacy more closely in Chapter 5.

However, another possibility is that reporting is better in hospitals. Perhaps it is less likely that a mistake will go unnoticed, because so many more people are involved in a patient's care. In the community, a patient may be seen by one doctor, one nurse, and perhaps one carer or family member, whereas in hospital it would not be unusual for twenty people to see that patient each day. On some days a patient in the community may not be seen at all, which is impossible in a hospital.

We have some additional information about medication incidents in primary care taken from the NPSA Quarterly Data Summary Issue 7. (NPSA, 2007(a): all NPSA reports are available from the website: **http://www.npsa.nhs.uk**.

The four most common areas for mistakes were vaccinations, prescribing (including errors made in generating the prescription), repeat prescribing and dispensing. Later in this chapter we will look at how each of these can be associated with mistakes, but you might like to pause for a moment to make your own list of suggestions.

The NPSA (2009) *Safety in Doses* report considered medication incidents across the whole field of healthcare, and noted some key lessons. The NPSA received 100 medication incident reports of death and severe harm via the NRLS in 2007: **http://www.nrls.npsa.nhs. uk/resources/?entryid45=61625**. Amongst these serious incidents, 41% were caused by errors in medicine administration and 32% by mistakes in prescribing. Injectable medicines led to 62% of all reports of death or severe harm. This is not surprising because a mistake involving an injection is more likely to involve a frail patient. In addition medicines used by injection act quite quickly and cannot be easily removed from the body once they have been administered, so errors are more likely to prove serious than with oral medication.

The analysis showed that nearly three-quarters of all incidents were caused by three types of error:

- The patient was given the wrong dose or was given it at the wrong time (for example, four times a day instead of two)
- The wrong medicine was given
- Doses which should have been given were missed or given late.

Obviously some medicines are more likely to cause harm than others, either because they are more dangerous in themselves or because they are given to patients who are critically ill. It is not surprising that among these are drugs which interfere with blood clotting or the action of the heart. Some medicines that have been associated with serious harms in the past have been the subject of special guidance from NPSA. Among these are methotrexate and potassium chloride. The fact that neither of these was linked to death or serious harm in patients in 2007 shows that if we try harder and take sensible precautions, we can reduce the incidence of harm. One key theme of this book is that we can all do better by thinking carefully about the way we do our jobs.

How can we reduce the incidence of harm from medication?

Most medication incidents do not cause any serious or lasting harm to the patient. This is true even if we do not take any action once they have happened. An example might be if a patient who has been prescribed the antibiotic amoxicillin in a 500 mg dose three times a day for seven days receives twenty 500 mg doses but one 250 mg dose by mistake.

Some incidents may lead to harm, but healthcare professionals are able to intervene to reduce the harm, perhaps by giving an antidote or stopping an infusion before it finishes.

There will be instances of serious harm which are unavoidable. Sometimes a carefully assessed risk is taken, with the agreement of the patient, because they have a serious medical condition. For example, an anti-cancer drug may cause harm. On other occasions, harm could not have been foreseen, either because the result was very unusual or because it arose from a factor peculiar to the individual. The muscle relaxant suxamethonium was used safely for a great many people but some patients died as a result of its use because they did not have the enzyme needed to break the drug down for elimination from their bodies. At the time there was no way of identifying them in advance.

However, that leaves a number of cases where the serious harm was avoidable. The NPSA/NRLS tries to understand what caused these events so that we can learn from them and take steps to reduce the chance that they will happen to patients in our care.

If we think carefully about how we use medication the number of errors can be reduced. The number of events will never reach zero; there will always be a few cases of harm when seriously ill patients have to be given powerful drugs, but we are a long way from that now.

The importance of near misses

The group described earlier—those where harm could have happened but was prevented by some sort of intervention—are sometimes described as near misses.

It is important that near misses are reported to NRLS, because they may give useful information about a problem. After all, they are 'near misses' because an error occurred. It does not stop being an error because someone put things right.

While a lot of near misses are reported to NRLS, it is very likely that many go unreported. There are good reasons for believing this to be the case. First, when nurses are asked to recall incidents they have seen or heard about, many will recall as many near misses as actual uncorrected errors (Myers et al, 2008). Second, our everyday experience in other areas tells us that near misses may be more common than accidents or mistakes. This suggests that there may be much more source material that we could use in our search for the cause of errors if we could reliably capture information on near misses. It is therefore important that nurses (and others) should report near misses in the same way as harmful incidents.

Sometimes healthcare professionals think that there is no need to report an incident that causes no harm, but this is quite wrong. It may happen again, and next time the patient may not be so lucky, or staff may react in the wrong way and fail to keep them safe. Another key reason is that outcome is not a proof of negligence. This is shown by comparing two scenarios. If you drink two bottles of wine and drive at high speed along a motorway, you may escape an accident, if only because others get out of your way. The fact that you survive does not mean that it was not reckless. On the other hand, there are many examples of people who have died through freak accidents in which no-one can be blamed. There, the outcome was very bad, but there was no negligence. If we only report bad outcomes, we will miss all those incidents that did not cause death or serious harm even though important mistakes may have been made. (Lamb and Nagpal, 2009)

Never events

Never events are serious events affecting patient safety which, on the whole, are preventable and should not have occurred if the available preventative measures were implemented. For more information on never events, please visit: **http://www.nrls.npsa.nhs.uk/neverevents/**.

What actions most commonly lead to mistakes?

As shown earlier, the commonest areas for mistakes were: vaccination, prescribing, repeat prescribing, and dispensing. If these are to be reduced additional information is needed to narrow down where the risks really are. NPSA has conducted this analysis on the data it holds, and the results for 2007 are shown in Figure 2.1.

NPSA suggests that the reason there are more reports of administration errors than other types is simply that more can go wrong at the point of giving a medicine to a patient.

If it is true that medicines management is giving the right dose of the right medicine at the right time to the right patient, then getting any of these wrong will constitute an error. During administration errors can be made in all of these. This is demonstrated in Figure 2.2.

Vaccination

There are a number of reasons why vaccinations may be particularly prone to error. Some of these have been identified by the National Patient Safety Agency in its reports (NPSA, 2007a).

First, vaccination clinics are frequently very busy and the nurses may be operating as sole workers—that is, they are undertaking all the care for a patient themselves. There is nobody else to provide a proper check on their actions. Second, in some clinics the great majority of those attending have come for the same vaccination, which makes it possible that a small number of those who need a different injection will be missed. Vaccines tend to have similar names—for example, there is little difference in name between two diphtheria, tetanus, pertussis and polio vaccines known as DTaP/IPV or dTaP/IPV, or indeed the similar vaccine which also covers *Haemophilus influenzae* type b, DTaP/IPV/Hib—and are often made by the same manufacturer who uses similar packaging. The

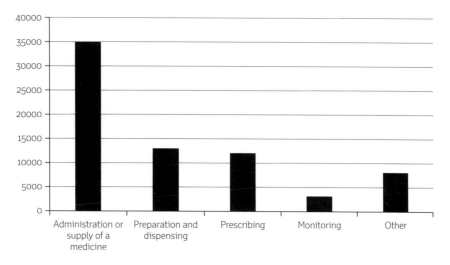

Figure 2.1 Number of incidents by stage of the medication process, 2007.
Safety in doses, NPSA, 2009.

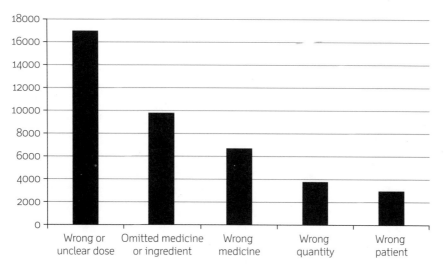

Figure 2.2 Number of medication incidents by error type, 2007.
Safety in doses, NPSA, 2009.

nurses at the clinic may not have full patient notes and may not be the patient's normal care providers, so they may not realise that they have confused two brothers, for example.

Another possible reason for mistakes is that the vaccination schedule for children changes from time to time. While nurses who work in these clinics often have a good grasp of the schedule, those who are infrequent vaccinators may not be so familiar with the correct ages and doses for vaccination. Clinics may be run in a range of settings where the nurse is unfamiliar with the

storage, the records, or the brands of vaccine used. This unfamiliarity adds to the stress in running a busy clinic.

Finally, the vaccine itself may not have been properly handled. Maintaining the cold chain (that is, ensuring that the vaccine stays refrigerated at all times from the factory to the clinic) can be complex and difficult. For example, the vaccine may be kept in a vaccine porter, which is a specialized cool box suitable for short periods of time. If someone forgets to replace the lid immediately after taking vaccine out, the temperature cannot be preserved and the vaccine may spoil.

Prescriptions

It is unlikely that pre-registration nurses will be involved in preparation of prescriptions, but we include this for completeness. There may be mistakes in the identity of the patient or the strength or dose of the medicines prescribed. It is possible that the prescriber will not know or may forget that a patient has a **contraindication** to a particular medicine (a contraindication is a reason why that medication is not suitable for them) or that they are already taking another medicine with which there will be an interaction. While nurses may rarely be in a position to make these mistakes, an alert nurse may notice that there has been an error and be able to intervene. Case studies 2.1, 2.2, and 2.3 will serve to demonstrate how errors can occur.

Consider how each of these might have been prevented. Notice that in each of these cases taken from real life it was a nurse who intervened to reduce harm to the patient.

Case study 2.1

Miss Scarlet telephoned her surgery to ask for a prescription for her elderly mother. The receptionist who took the call passed a handwritten note to the duty doctor. Either it was unclear, or he misread it, but he issued a handwritten prescription for Miss Scarlet herself. Since she had the same surname as her mother, and the prescriber had not included the date of birth, Miss Scarlet did not know that the doctor had prescribed for a 50-year-old woman rather than her mother, who was in her eighties and rather frail. The older lady took the tablets until a visiting community nurse noticed them and queried the dose with the prescriber.

Case study 2.2

A resident in a care home providing nursing services was prescribed a high-carbohydrate feed by a doctor who was not aware that she suffered from diabetes. The nurse who collected the prescription questioned it with the pharmacist before it was dispensed, as a result an alternative choice was made.

Case study 2.3

A doctor intended to prescribe long-acting morphine tablets 10 mg to a patient, but selected the wrong item from the drop-down list on the surgery computer, with the result that a prescription for 100 mg was printed. The prescription was signed and dispensed, but at a later stage a nurse questioned why a patient had been started on such a high dose. There is now NPSA guidance requiring nurses to question large increases in the dosage of opiate painkillers.

Repeat prescribing

General practices operate a repeat prescription system whereby patients who regularly need the same medication can select it from a pre-printed list. This list should be reviewed at intervals to ensure that all the medication on it is still needed; otherwise a medicine that has been discontinued could be re-prescribed after a period of time (NPSA, 2007b).

Another potential problem occurs when a medicine was not being used when something else was prescribed, and the original doctor did not intend it to be prescribed again, but it is subsequently provided on a repeat prescription. An example may help to explain this. The antibiotic erythromycin is sometimes used for a period of months to treat cases of acne. When it is given alongside the antiepileptic drug carbamazepine, erythromycin slows down the metabolism of carbamazepine so that the level of that medicine in the patient's blood will rise, perhaps causing adverse effects. Dr A knew this, so when his patient needed carbamazepine he told the patient to stop taking the erythromycin that had previously been prescribed. Unfortunately it was not removed from her repeat list, so at a later date, when Dr A was on holiday, Dr B prescribed it again. If he had prescribed both erythromycin and carbamazepine at the same time, the practice computer would have drawn his attention to the error, but because Dr B only prescribed erythromycin the computer did not check for an interaction. (This is unusual; most systems would check against medicines that may still be in use).

Dispensing or administration

Strictly, dispensing refers to the preparation of the patient's medicines according to the prescription and is therefore usually done by pharmacists, whereas administration is the act of giving the medicine to the patient. Some patients will be able to look after their own medicines, whereas others may need help or support to take them.

The likely errors at this stage can be predicted. If the aim is to give the right dose of the right drug at the right time to the right patient, and any one of those can go wrong, attention must be paid to all four points at each administration. In everyday speech we sometimes quote Murphy's Law—if anything can go wrong, eventually it will—which reminds us that there is no mistake that cannot be made if we do not guard against it.

Exercise 2.1

> Before reading on, think how you could reduce the risk of error when giving a tablet to a patient on a hospital ward.

Right patient

Many care homes attach a photograph of each person to their medication record sheets to aid identification. Do not rely on their appearance alone—they may have a twin!—or on where you find them. They may be sitting on another person's bed. Confused patients, or those who are hard of hearing, may answer to someone else's name. Hospitals provide patients with named wristbands and there will be an identification procedure used wherever you work to ensure that you have the right patient for whatever you are going to do. This procedure must always be followed.

Right time

Sometimes the timing of a dose is critical. Antiviral drugs and those used in Parkinson's disease must be taken at regular intervals and therefore it is important that these should be given at the set times. In some cases it may not be the time on the clock that is important, but the time in relation to other treatment. For example, two anti-cancer drugs may have to be given in a particular order with a set time interval between them. A further complication is that some medicines must be taken before meals, whereas others are given after food. This may mean that you have to return to the same patient twice during a medicines round to ensure that these are given at the best times. If this happens there should be a procedure to make sure that the medicines that are given after meals are not forgotten.

Right drug

It is not enough to read the label on the medicine and compare it to the medicine chart, though this is essential. Nurses should become familiar with at least the most common medications they administer so that their appearance can be compared to what is expected. Appearance may differ from hospital to hospital according to the brands of tablets used there, but it should rarely change from day to day. If the local brand of the anti-inflammatory medicine naproxen is a long, yellow tablet, but on another day the same strength is a round, white tablet, the alert nurse will want to make further checks. In this case it may be that the long, yellow tablet is a 500 mg tablet while the round, white one is a 250 mg tablet, so the dispensing labels may explain the difference.

Right dose

In community practice, prescribers will normally express the dose in numbers of tablets, capsules, or 5 ml spoonsful of a given strength, thus:

> Tabs erythromycin 250 mg × 20
> Give TWO tablets twice a day for 5 days.

In hospitals it is not unusual to find the total dose given but not how the dose is made up. This example might be written:

> Erythromycin 500 mg twice a day for 5 days.

The nurse who gives the medication will have to check the dose of the tablets in the medicines trolley against the prescribed dose, and must not assume that the dose is always one tablet or capsule.

There may also be a limit on the total dose in 24 hours that must be observed. The maximum daily dose of paracetamol is usually eight 500 mg tablets, but it is quite common to see prescriptions for 'one or two tablets, up to four-hourly'. If the patient asks for two tablets every four hours, they will have 12 in a day, which is too many. In this case, it is not enough for nurses to initial the medicines chart to show that they have given a dose, because the next nurse will not know whether one tablet or two tablets were given earlier. Each nurse will have to note how many tablets were given at each dose.

This example also offers another reason for mistakes. There is a big difference between giving tablets 'four-hourly' and 'four hourly'. If you have any doubt what the prescriber meant, you must ask before giving the medication. The person who wrote an instruction knows what is meant and usually can only interpret it their way; the idea that it can be read in any other way may not have occurred to them. For example, how should we read this prescription for an antidiabetic tablet?

Gliclazide tablets 80 mg × 30
Give 1/2 every morning.

In this case, a nurse could read it as an instruction to give half a tablet each morning. In fact, the doctor meant one or two. The result could be that the patient was under-dosed. While the doctor can be criticized for not being clear, the nurse has a responsibility to question what was meant.

Increasingly hospitals use coloured wristbands to identify patients who have an allergy to a drug. The wristband—usually red—should alert nurses to the fact that an allergy has been noted in the patient's record, making it less likely that a nurse will not notice this when giving the medication.

Reason's Swiss cheese model of errors

Professor James Reason is a psychologist who has written extensively on the detection and prevention of errors. The summary which follows is only a small part of his work. Interested readers can find much more in his books such as *Human Error* (1990) and his many journal articles.

The Greek playwright Aeschylus is sometimes said to have been killed by a tortoise which was dropped on his head by a passing eagle (Healey, 1991). Whether it is true or not, it is plainly a very unlikely occurrence. The same thing could happen to any of us, but preventing it would probably mean that we would have to wear a crash helmet whenever we were outside. When we balance the risk of these very unlikely events against the inconvenience of the measures we need to take to avoid them, we may decide just to accept the small risk.

Reason noted that when risks are very small, we may become fatalistic about them, assuming that there is nothing practical that we can do to make them any less likely. We may fall into the trap of thinking of these events as rather like lightning strikes, completely unpredictable and unavoidable. In fact, he said, if we analyse them properly, even rare incidents can be seen to have a definite probability and it may be possible to reduce that even further.

In his Swiss cheese model, Reason gave us an analogy (see Figure 2.3).

Reason suggested that the barriers we put in the way of errors—protocols, drills, physical measures such as locks or swipe cards, for example—are not perfect. They are rather like slices of Swiss cheese. Accidents happen when all the barriers fail at the same time. In

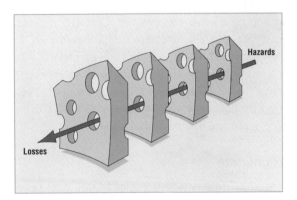

Figure 2.3 Reason's Swiss Cheese model of error. Reproduced from *BMJ* 2000; 320: 768–770 with permission of BMJ Publishing Ltd.

his analogy, he shows such an event as the moment when the holes in the cheese line up so the arrow can pass through them.

If a measure is 98% effective, that is rather like saying that a slice of cheese consists of 2% holes. If we have four such measures, as in the diagram, the chances that a potential error can pass through all four slices would be 0.02 × 0.02 × 0.02 × 0.02 or 0.000 000 16. That means that there would be 16 chances in 100 million that this event would happen. Even though this is very unlikely, the model says that it can (and probably will) happen sometime, but the model also shows us how we could make it less likely. We could improve each slice of the cheese so that it had smaller holes, or we could introduce more slices. If we halve the number of holes in one slice, we halve the risk overall; halve the risk in all four slices, and risk is divided by 16 to one in 100 million. If we can add a fifth slice like the others we reduce the risk to 2% of what it was—that is, fifty times smaller. Even if we do not know the exact percentage of holes in each slice, we can see how we could improve matters.

If we translate this to our study of medical errors, we can see its application quite readily. Suppose that a doctor makes a mistake in writing a prescription. In order for that error to harm the patient, it would have to avoid detection by the dispenser in the pharmacy, the pharmacist who checks the dispensed medicine, and the nurse who gave it to the patient. If we add a check by a second nurse, the risk is immediately reduced again, provided that the second nurse really performs their own check and does not just rely on their colleague having checked it. If a nurse does not carry out their own independent check, they may as well not be there.

In this example of a prescribing error, there would be four slices of cheese to trap the mistake—a dispenser, a pharmacist and two nurses. Obviously an error made by a nurse in giving the medicine to the patient only has to pass one slice (a second nurse who checks). That is one reason why errors in administration are relatively common.

Since each slice of cheese reduces risk, you might ask why we do not keep adding slices until all the risks are gone. There are two reasons. First, each check slows down the process of getting medicine to the patient, and while we should make time for necessary checks, there comes a point at which we cannot fit in more checks without hampering patient care. Second, there is some evidence that when we know someone else is going to check further down the line, we may become a little less careful, so adding more checks may not produce the whole improvement that we expect.

Since we are all human beings, and humans make mistakes, no barrier to error that depends on us will ever be completely free of holes. However, machinery is much less prone to error. Mechanical or computerized checks offer the possibility of producing slices with much smaller holes, or indeed no holes at all. The NPSA report *Design for patient safety* (NPSA 2007c) gives a number of examples of safety enhancements brought about by use of computerization. For example, in some dispensaries the barcode on the boxes of tablets is scanned by the dispenser so the drug name automatically appears on the dispensing label, reducing the risk that the wrong medicine will be typed in. The same principle is beginning to be used on some wards, where nurses can scan a barcode on a container and see what should be on the medication chart. If there is a mismatch they can make enquiries. One of the early successes of NPSA was in altering the connectors on injections given into the space around the spinal cord to make it impossible to connect the wrong type of syringe. There had been several incidents of very toxic anti-cancer drugs being wrongly injected into the epidural space in this way (Toft, 2001), but since the introduction of syringes for this use with a specialized connector, it is much more difficult to make this mistake.

Another example, which has yet to be implemented, involves access to cabinets containing controlled drugs such as morphine. At present, a key is needed, which should be securely stored at all times. However, anyone who finds the key could access the cabinet. It is possible to produce smart cards for staff such that their hospital identity card would include a code that allowed them to open the cabinet, and would record who did it. The system could even automatically telephone the ward if the cabinet seemed to have been left open.

However, important though technology may be, it does not absolve healthcare professionals from the need to take all the care they can in using medication. Accepting that humans make mistakes is not the same as thinking that mistakes are themselves acceptable. Reason addresses this in another important strand of work (see, for example, Reason, 2000).

There are two approaches to the management of error. Reason calls one the person approach and the other the system approach. The person approach requires each individual to try constantly to improve their performance, and blames them for any lapses or mistakes that they make because potentially we can all do better. It sees the causes of mistakes as being lapses in concentration, forgetfulness, or recklessness, all of which we could avoid if we tried harder. This is the approach that has long been followed in the NHS, and the way in which those who follow it try to reduce human error is to retrain people, to run poster campaigns threatening people with the consequences of their errors, and treating errors as blameworthy incidents just because they happened. Reason describes this in the article as a culture of 'naming, blaming, and shaming' (2000). He also notes that it assumes that we deserve blame because bad things happen to bad people. Accidents do not 'just happen'; they happen because we make bad decisions.

An alternative approach is to accept that humans cannot perform perfectly over the longer term and that mistakes will therefore happen, so the key is to put systems in place that reduce reliance on individuals and shield patients from the consequences of mistakes. In this analysis, errors are seen not as events that humans create, but as the result of pressures put on us from imperfections in the system. If we improve the system, we can change the environment in which people work so that there is less pressure on them and a reduced chance of error.

This also changes the reporting culture in an organization. If it adopts the people approach, nurses who make mistakes may try to hide them because they do not want to be blamed. Since nobody hears that a particular type of mistake has been made, no steps will be taken to stop it happening again, so it is likely to be repeated.

Let us consider a scenario. It was difficult for various reasons for nurses to get the medicine trolley into a two-bedded bay in a community hospital because a table which was fixed to the wall was in the way. Nurses found it difficult to push the medicines trolley past it and turn in at the adjoining doorway that led to the two-bedded bay. They therefore fell into the habit of putting those patients' medications into unmarked cups before walking the last few metres to the bedside.

One day a nurse accidentally muddled the cups and the two residents received each other's medication. No harm resulted, but the nurse said nothing about it because they were afraid of being disciplined. As a result, nurses went on transferring medicines into unmarked cups and no changes were made. It would obviously have been better if the nurses had taken the labelled pack of tablets to the bedside. This problem could have been avoided if there had been the space to take the medicine trolley to the patients. If the nurse who had made the first error had reported it then problems could have been identified and similar incidents could have been prevented.

This example illustrates the benefits of the system approach. If those who are investigating are not looking for someone to blame, but instead focus on the way that things are done and how that allows mistakes to happen, they may see where the real problem lies. In the people approach, each incident is examined in isolation to see who was to blame for that event. In the systems approach, investigators look for patterns and linkages, so they are more likely to find continuing causes of errors. Mistakes are not random events. They happen for a reason, and it is easier to see a reason when you do not treat each occurrence as a one-off mistake.

Again, an example may help. There have been examples of pharmacists intending to dispense two identical packs, but accidentally picking up two drugs for two different conditions because the two packs sat next to each other in alphabetical order and were therefore side by side on the shelf. Tablets often also come in similar coloured boxes as was the case for the above drugs. Under a person approach, the enquiry would have been directed towards finding out which pharmacist made the mistake and telling them to take more care in future. That might reduce the risk that the same person would do it again, but it does not prevent other people making that mistake. The system approach might suggest that the packs should be bought from different suppliers so they look different, and should be separated on the shelves. Accordingly, it is now best practice to keep tablets for the different conditions in a separate part of the dispensary shelving.

NB: NPSA 2007(d) guidance is that manufacturers who produce drugs with similar names within their range distinguish between them by using different coloured packaging.

For further reading regarding scenarios and safety recommendations from the NPSA please access the following link: **http://www.nrls.npsa.nhs.uk/EasySite-Web/getresource.axd?AssetID=63052&type=full&servicetype=Attachment**.

Active failures and latent conditions

Reason explains that the two approaches detect different types of problems. Active failures are the things that nurses and others do at the bedside. They are the immediate acts that lead to a risk of harm. Some of them may not be mistakes as we would normally use that word. They may be deliberate decisions that just work out badly. A consistent finding in inquiries is that healthcare professionals make choices that introduce risk, sometimes for reasons that seem good to them at the time and often designed to help the patient. For example, a nurse might give a painkilling injection without a check from a second nurse rather than leaving their patient in pain until someone is free. That is certainly an active failure but it can hardly be described as accidental if the nurse deliberately chose to do it.

Latent conditions are the underlying problems that will probably surface one day by causing untoward events. To use a common term, they are the bugs in the system. They are always there but they only lead to accidents when they are paired with an active failure.

Examples of latent conditions might include staff shortages, failure to maintain important equipment, time pressure, inadequate training, or forcing people to multitask during their working day. The person approach to fault-finding will not track down latent conditions systematically, because the inquiry will stop when it finds an active failure that explains what happened. The systems approach, however, has a much better chance of uncovering a latent condition so it can be corrected before an incident occurs.

The system approach in action

A fine example of this approach in use was provided by Professor Brian Toft's enquiry (2001) following the unfortunate death of Wayne Jowett. Professor Toft's report can be read at: **http://www.dh.gov.uk/en/Publicationsandstatistics/Publications/PublicationsPolicyAndGuidance/DH_4010064**.

Wayne Jowett was receiving chemotherapy for leukaemia as a day case patient at a hospital in the Midlands. This treatment involved giving one medicine by intrathecal injection (into the space around the spinal cord) while another anticancer drug, vincristine, was given intravenously. A senior house officer was given this to do, and although supervised by a specialist registrar, he gave both medicines intrathecally. Vincristine given in this way is usually fatal, and so it proved here. Despite prompt emergency treatment, Mr Jowett died nearly a month later.

Professor Toft's report described five immediate or active failures, some of which fell far short of good practice. However, he went on to say, 'The evidence presented to this inquiry suggests that the adverse incident that led to Mr Jowett's death was not caused by one or even several human errors but by a far more complex amalgam of human, organizational, technical, and social interactions . . .' and to list 39 latent conditions that contributed to the accident. His response to these factors was to suggest 56 recommendations for improvement.

A person approach would probably have been satisfied when no less than five reasons for the accident were detected and the culprits identified. However, that would not have addressed most of the 39 other reasons that Professor Toft identified, some of which were not unique to the hospital involved but were helpful in avoiding incidents across the country.

Some of the causes that Professor Toft describes should have been clear to any sensible observer, and an astute nurse might have suggested changes that could have prevented the accident. For example, although there was an elaborate system to bring the two injections to the ward by separate routes at different times to prevent confusion, when they arrived on the ward they were placed on the same shelf in the same refrigerator. Someone might have asked why such a complicated procedure was in place if it made no difference in the end. Despite the presence of hazardous medicines, the refrigerator was unlocked and there were no restrictions on access, so any nurse could collect the injections. Although nursing staff were aware that two different versions of the same haematology guideline were on the ward, nobody had reported this to their line manager so the old version could be destroyed. This report emphasizes that patient safety is everyone's concern; all healthcare professionals can make a difference if they understand the principles involved in analysing risks.

Wider application

In the example just quoted, it was remarked that the findings from this inquiry improved practice across the country. This can be true of a lot of patient safety initiatives.

A simple example may illustrate this. Errors in medicines administration can occur when nurses are interrupted. It is not unusual for patients who are given their tablets to choose that moment to ask for a bedpan. This disturbance can increase the risk of errors, particularly in calculations.

In some areas, nurses conducting medicines rounds are given a tabard labelled, 'Please do not disturb me', or coloured tabards and instructed not to answer telephones or leave the round until they have finished.

Even if tabards are not appropriate, there must be occasions when it is important that healthcare workers are not disturbed. No one would want to hear of surgeons answering their mobile phones during an operation, for example. When pharmacists are filling monitored dosage systems (boxes which hold patients' tablets and capsules in a date and time layout so all

the tablets given together are in one blister) it is easy to lose their place if they are distracted. Readers may be able to think of other occasions when it is important that they should not be disturbed.

Using guidelines and protocols to reduce risks

Unfortunately, much of health care cannot be automated. If we have to rely on human beings, how can we reduce their errors?

One possibility can be seen by looking at the natural path of a career. When we are young, we know relatively little about our career, and need to be supervised. In time, our performance improves and, we hope, will continue to improve with experience. There may come a time when our work declines because we are ageing, but, in general, we get better with experience.

We are also aware that a group of people is less likely to make a mistake than a single person. That is not to say that it will never happen, but the whole point of having two nurses check a dose when giving a controlled drug (NMC, 2010) is that it is less likely that two will make a mistake than one will. Sadly, we cannot go about our daily work in groups.

However, we can put these two ideas together. How can we pass experience from the old to the young so that the young student can learn faster? And how can we give everyone the support of a group which is not actually with them all the time?

The answer is that we can get a group of experienced people to write protocols or guidelines. These words are often used interchangeably, but there is a slight difference. A guideline gives a general direction, but allows for variations. The National Institute for Health and Clinical Excellence (NICE) says that its guidelines are likely to cover around 80% of patients at best (NICE, 2001) so the guideline must allow some options for the remaining 20%. A protocol, however, is a strict description of a way of doing things; in diplomacy, for example, a protocol describes the only way that something should be carried out. (Concise Oxford English Dictionary, 2008)

Guidelines and protocols allow us to learn from the collected experience of others. By setting out the majority view on how best to perform a task, a guideline gives us a standard to work to. In the field of safety, one common type of protocol is the checklist. Sometimes healthcare professionals object to having to complete a checklist repeatedly because they feel that it belittles their skill as a professional, but when we fly abroad on holiday we hope our pilot is a skilled professional yet we would be unhappy if he ignored the pre-flight checklist and relied on his experience to spot any problems with the aeroplane.

Used properly, checklists can make great differences. Merry (2001) gives the example of an anaesthetic department in New Zealand which improved sharply after introducing checklists for anaesthetic machines to ensure that they were properly set up before operations. The World Health Organization has also endorsed checklists (Humphreys, 2008). A multinational trial showed that following a nineteen-point checklist before non-cardiac surgery reduced the death rate by almost half (Haynes, 2009). One member of that group has published a book which gives more evidence for the usefulness of checklists (Gawande, 2010).

In healthcare, there are two variations on checklists that keep some of the benefits of a checklist but may be better suited to our practice. Instead of a written checklist, we may have a drill, which is a specified series of actions, perhaps with spoken instructions. For example, it would be difficult to break off while resuscitating a patient to tick a checklist, but it is still important that everyone involved should know what they have to do and when. Almost every type of emergency treatment is likely to use drills rather than a written list. Most of us learned to cross the road as children by using a drill, such as the kerb drill:

- Stand where you can clearly see both ways
- Look right
- Look left
- Look right again
- If all is clear, walk straight across
- Keep looking!

In the context of medicines management, there may be drills for checking the drugs stock, deciding the route around the ward, describing how medicines are given to the patient (in the order they are written on the chart, for example), when the paperwork is to be completed, how to record a refusal by a patient to take a medicine, and so on.

Increasingly, these drills are captured on paper as standard operating procedures (SOPs, pronounced by the initials or as 'sops'). SOPs follow a standard local format—so they may differ from place to place, but usually are similar within one area—and describe how something should be done. They are not usually intended to be read as the action they describe is performed. Instead, we read them beforehand and learn how to follow them, perhaps by performing trial runs under supervision. A SOP describes in detail what equipment needs to be gathered before you start, what forms will need to be completed, and every step that must be followed to complete the task.

Exercise 2.2

> To illustrate how these are written, we can try writing one for an everyday task.
> Before reading on, write a set of instructions to tell someone how to make a pot of tea.

The SOP you produce may not be the same as someone else's, but it would be possible for a group to agree one between them that showed their idea of the best way to make tea. Our SOP for tea-making would include:

- The equipment needed—teapot, kettle, and spoon
- The ingredients—teabags, milk, sugar, drinkable water (if you only put 'water', your reader might take it from a muddy puddle)
- A simple description of all the steps needed to make tea in the correct order including the number of teabags needed and the time to leave the tea to brew.

Individual nurses will not be asked to write procedures such as these, but as you gain experience you may be asked to help by reviewing or writing an SOP for an area of your expertise.

Learning from our mistakes

One key instruction of the Nursing and Midwifery Council's Code (2008) is that nurses should always practise within their limits of competence. Unfortunately the psychologists Justin Kruger and David Dunning showed that those of us who are incompetent are also very bad at recognizing that we are incompetent (Kruger and Dunning, 1999). Dunning has published several papers since with a similar theme, and has particularly noted the challenge for health professionals that this Kruger–Dunning effect (the inability to detect your own incompetence) may bring.

One answer that is proposed to this problem is not to let people assess their own competence, but to make them prove it to others. In order that the examination should be fair and comprehensive, the tasks are broken down into simple competences and students illustrate each one in turn. A description of the process can be found in an article by Strasser et al (2005).

When a mistake occurs, the competences that each healthcare professional believes they have can be re-examined and, perhaps, re-tested. If, for example, they have miscalculated a dose, is this an isolated mistake or have they forgotten how a particular calculation is done? Even if nobody formally re-tests us, we should be prepared to re-examine ourselves. One of the important findings of Dunning's work has been that people who are interested in improving their skills are less likely to overstate their competence than those who show no interest in going forward in their careers.

Significant event analysis

Just as individuals can re-examine practice in the light of an error, so can organizations or teams. This can be done informally, but better results are obtained by conducting a formal analysis of the case, called a significant event analysis (SEA).

The Toft report (2001) into the death of Wayne Jowett was essentially a very big significant event analysis. It gathered all the evidence it could, tested it to see who was telling the truth and who was mistaken, tried to put together a detailed description of what went wrong, then examined each step carefully to see what might have been done differently.

NHS Education for Scotland has a useful toolkit for conducting a significant event analysis (SEA) on its website at: **http://www.scottishappraisal.scot.nhs.uk/ toolkit/good-clinical-care-(gp-scot-1b)/significant-event-analysis.aspx**.

The toolkit illustrates that a successful SEA contains seven steps.

1 Identify and prioritize the significant event. How important is it?

2 Collect the facts. What happened exactly? Who was there? Who could give us evidence?

3 Arrange a meeting to discuss. Bring people together who can give evidence and some outsiders who know the best questions to ask to gain an understanding of what happened. For example, if there is a problem on a ward, it may be helpful to ask a ward manager from another hospital to describe what they would have done to see if your local habits are not best practice.

4 Undertake a structured analysis. Be logical about breaking the event into the smallest possible steps and examine each in turn, looking for improvements that could be made.

5 Monitor agreed change. If you have made changes you think will improve matters, little is gained until you have checked that they really have made a difference.

6 Write it up. The evidence you have may help someone elsewhere to avoid an incident, so you have a professional duty to share your new learning. Until it is shared, patients elsewhere are still at risk.

7 Peer review. If you have confidence that you have made improvements these should be clear to colleagues. Allow them to examine what has happened to see if the changes are lasting and worthwhile.

Serious untoward incident policies

NHS organizations will have policies on how to handle serious untoward incidents (SUIs, often pronounced as 'soo-ees'). There is sometimes confusion about the relationship between an SUI and an SEA.

The SUI is the accident or mistake that takes place and the SUI policy should describe how and to whom it should be reported. It may also describe how the ward or unit should react in the immediate aftermath of the incident. For example, it may say that if there is an incident in an operating theatre, that theatre cannot be used until an inspection has taken place.

The SEA is the inquiry into the accident or mistake that tries to find causes and remedies for it. Since the SUI is the trigger for an SEA, some departments have a policy which includes instructions for setting up an SEA as part of their SUI policy since both will be needed for the same event, but strictly the two are separate responses to it. Sometimes these have to be separated, because the SEA has to be led by a specified person. For example, the unexpected death of a patient may be a SUI, but the investigation into the death (an SEA) may have to be led by the coroner or procurator fiscal.

The national reporting and learning system (NRLS) and the yellow card system

Some responses to events have to be made in a particular way. The NPSA's national reporting and learning system consists of a user-friendly website form that asks appropriate questions based upon the way that other questions are answered. For example, if you say that the incident took place on a hospital ward, the software hides all the questions about a dispensary so you need not answer those.

The website is not the only way that information can be gathered for NRLS, and some Trusts or Health Boards have an internal reporting system that means that a person or department makes all the reports for that hospital or unit. The Trust has a form or report that is completed, then, when the information has been checked and is as complete as possible, it is relayed to NRLS.

The law requires that incidents concerning controlled drugs must be reported to the organization's accountable officer for controlled drugs. This is usually done by your line manager, but if the accountable officer (AO) needs a report or has questions, they may

contact you directly. The AO carries the responsibility for the organization's safe use of controlled drugs and when something may have gone amiss they must take immediate steps to ensure patient safety. This might mean that they tell you to stay behind after your shift, or come in on a day off to answer questions. If this happens, it is not because they think you are at fault. It happens because they have to complete their inquiries very quickly. When a serious incident occurs, the AO's team may work non-stop until they are sure that there is no further risk to patients.

Another specified system exists for reporting adverse effects to medicines. This is the yellow card reporting system, so called because originally reports were made on yellow postcards. An example of such a card can be seen at the back of each copy of the *British National Formulary*. These reports are forwarded to the Medicines and Healthcare products Regulatory Agency (MHRA) which licenses medicines and collates reports of their side effects. There is now a website through which reports can be made: **http://yellowcard.mhra.gov.uk/**, which also contains more information about how the scheme works.

Anyone can make a report to MHRA but to avoid duplication caused by a number of health workers sending in their own reports of the same incident, some organizations specify who will make reports. This might be the chief pharmacist or the medical director, for example.

Personal accountability

Personal accountability was introduced in Chapter 1, but here we examine how it applies in medicines management.

Student and registered nurses are personally accountable for the way in which they administer medicines (NMC, 2010, 2011a) if that task has been delegated to them by a registered nurse. If you have doubts about your competence to fulfil this role, then you discharge your duty of accountability by making your concerns known to the nurse in charge. The registered nurse should not delegate any job to a student who has not demonstrated their competence; the registered nurse's own accountability means that they should be satisfied that the student is able to perform the delegated work properly (NMC, 2008).

This is also true when you can perform most of the role, but not all of it. For example, you may be competent to give tablets and capsules, but not have trained to give injections or suppositories. In this case you may carry out the administration of oral doses, but would explain to the delegating nurse that you are not yet ready to take on the other tasks.

Sometimes students think that observing someone else does not need any particular competence. That is generally true, but it does not apply to being a second checker. Generally where two nurses have different degrees of competence, the more competent nurse should check medicines rather than administer them. However, strict application of this rule would mean that students would never learn to act as second checkers, because their mentor would always fill that role. In no circumstances should a nurse who is not competent to perform a duty undertake to check someone else doing it without having been trained to perform that particular check (NMC, 2008). This is particularly true of the administration of controlled drugs. Having said this, checking a more senior colleague's administration of medicines can be a good introduction to medicines management provided that you are clear what you are checking and why. If you are not clear why you are being asked to check something, say so.

Finally, we all have a duty to report any errors or incidents that come to our notice, even if we did not make them (and even if we do not know who did). It can be difficult to report a mistake that has been made by a friend or colleague, but our accountability must extend to protecting patients at all times and in all circumstances (CQC, 2011; NMC, 2011b). Equally, if the mistake is ours, we must report it, or we place our colleagues in the awkward position of having to report our mistake for us.

Summary

Patient safety is everyone's concern. Our first duty is not to harm our patient and since medication can cause harm, we must be careful in its use. When mistakes are made we must see that they are honestly reported so that we can learn from our mistakes and help colleagues not to make the same mistakes. Following procedures, drills, or protocols can reduce the number of errors we make.

References

Care Quality Commission (2011) *Raising a Concern with CQC: A Quick Guide for Health and Care Staff*. Available at: http://www.nmc-uk.org/Press-and-media/Latest-news/CQC-publishes-new-guide-on-whistleblowing/ (accessed 16 December 2012).

Concise Oxford English Dictionary (2008). Oxford: Oxford University Press.

Department of Health (2010), *Equity and Excellence: Liberating the NHS*. London: TSO.

Gawande A (2010), *The Checklist Manifesto: How to get things right*. London: Profile Books.

Haynes AB, Weiser TG, Berry WR, Lipsitz SR, Breizat AS, Dellinger P, et al (2009). A surgical safety checklist to reduce morbidity and mortality in a global population, *New England Journal of Medicine*, 360; 491–499.

Healey J (ed) (1991), *Natural History by Secundius Gaisus Pliny the Elder*. London: Penguin Books.

Humphreys G (2008), Checklists save lives. *Bulletin of the World Health Organization*, 86; 501–502.

Kruger J and Dunning D (1999), Unskilled and Unaware of It: How difficulties in recognizing one's own incompetence lead to inflated self-assessments, *Journal of Personality and Social Psychology*, 77; 1121–1134.

Lamb BW and Nagpal K (2009), Importance of near misses, *British Medical Journal*, 339; b3032.

Merry A (2001), *Errors, Medicine and the Law*. Cambridge: Cambridge University Press, p 123.

Myers JA, Dominici F, and Morlock L (2008), Learning from near misses in medication errors: a Bayesian approach (December 2008). *Johns Hopkins University, Dept. of Biostatistics Working Papers*. Working Paper 178. Available at: http://www.bepress.com/jhubiostat/paper178 (accessed 16 December 2012).

National Institute for Clinical Excellence (2001), *Response to the Report of the Bristol Royal Infirmary Inquiry*. Available at: http://www.nice.org.uk/niceMedia/pdf/bristolreportresponsefinal.pdf (accessed 16 December 2012).

National Patient Safety Agency (2007a), *Quarterly Data Summary Issue 7: Medication Incidents in Primary Care*. Available at: http://www.nrls.npsa.nhs.uk/resources/?EntryId45=59839 (accessed 16 December 2012).

National Patient Safety Agency (2007b), PSO/4: *Safety in Doses: Medication Safety Incidents in the NHS*. Available at: http://www.nrls.npsa.nhs.uk/resources/?entryid45=61625 (accessed 16 December 2012).

National Patient Safety Agency (2007c), Available at: http://www.nrls.npsa.nhs.uk/resources/collections/design-for-patient-safety/ (accessed 16 December 2012).

National Patient Safety Agency (2007d), *Design for Patient Safety: A Guide to the Graphic Design of Medication Packaging*. 2nd ed. Available at: http://www.nrls.npsa.nhs.uk/EasySiteWeb/getresource.axd?AssetID=63052&type=full&servicetype=Attachment (accessed 16 December 2012).

National Patient Safety Agency (2009), *Safety in Doses: Improving the Use of Medicines in the NHS*. Available at: http://www.nrls.npsa.nhs.uk/resources/?entryid45=61625 (accessed 16 December 2012).

NHS Litigation Authority (2011), *Annual Report and Accounts*. Available at: http://www.official-documents.gov.uk/document/hc1012/hc11/1113/1113.pdf (accessed 16 December 2012).

Nursing and Midwifery Council (2008), *The Code of Conduct, Performance and Ethics*. London: NMC.

Nursing and Midwifery Council (2010), *Standards for Medicines Management*. London: NMC.

Nursing and Midwifery Council (2011a), *Guidance on Professional Conduct for Nursing and Midwifery Students*. London: NMC.

Nursing and Midwifery Council (2011b), *Raising Escalating Concerns*. London: NMC.

Reason J (1990), *Human Error*. Cambridge: Cambridge University Press.

Reason J (2000), Human error: models and management, *British Medical Journal* 320: 768–770.

Strasser S, London L, and Kortenbout E (2005), Developing a competence framework and evaluation tool for primary care nursing in South Africa, *Education for Health*, 18; 133–144.

Toft B (2001), *External Inquiry into the Adverse Incident that occurred at Queen's Medical Centre, Nottingham, 4th January 2001*, Department of Health. Available at http://www.dh.gov.uk/en/Publicationsandstatistics/Publications/PublicationsPolicyAndGuidance/DH_4010064 (Accessed 16 December 2012).

3 Principles of Pharmacology

CHAPTER CONTENTS

- Basic pharmacokinetics
- Absorption
- Distribution
- Metabolism
- Excretion
- Key pharmacokinetic concepts
- Pharmacogenetics
- Pharmacodynamics
- Adverse drug reactions
- Drug interactions
- Quiz
- Complementary medicines
- Summary

LEARNING OUTCOMES

After reading this chapter, you should be able to:

- Understand the pharmacological aspects of drugs
- Understand the concepts of pharmacokinetics, pharmacodynamics, and pharmacogenetics
- Understand what is meant by the pharmacokinetic phases of absorption, distribution, metabolism, and excretion and describe how drugs pass through the body during these phases
- Understand first pass metabolism and how it may be reduced
- Understand the terms 'half-life', 'bioavailability', and 'therapeutic window'
- Describe how genetics affects an individual's ability to metabolize medicines
- Distinguish between the first and second phases of liver metabolism
- Give an account of the lock and key hypothesis in drug-receptor interactions
- Explain, and distinguish between, agonists, antagonists, and partial agonists
- Explain why adverse drug reactions are often predictable
- Understand and classify drug interactions.

From the previous chapters you will see that understanding the pharmacological aspects of the drugs you are administering is vital to keeping your patients safe.

Box 3.1 Why do nurses need to know about pharmacology?

To predict and understand adverse reactions and interactions and thereby keep patients safe.

To understand why different medicines are given at varying intervals and in varying doses.

To support patients in getting the maximum benefit from their treatment by ensuring that they receive the right dose of the right medicine and understand what their medicine is intended to do.

Nurses need to understand the pharmacodynamics of a medicine, or how it actually works within the body, since this will need to be explained to patients and carers. For example, how will you ensure that a patient understands the importance of taking their treatment for hypertension (especially if they are experiencing no symptoms) if you are unable to explain how the medicine will be working?

Similarly, your understanding of the pharmacokinetics (the absorption, distribution, metabolism, and excretion) of individual medicines is vital to ensure compromised patients are not administered inappropriate medicines. For example, you would question the prescribing of a non-steroidal anti-inflammatory drug (NSAID) to a patient with significant renal impairment, because the kidney is essential to the elimination of NSAIDs so the drug could accumulate if the kidneys are not functioning properly.

From the point of view of ensuring patient safety, you will need to understand the principles of drug interactions so that you can understand how two medicines (or food and medicine) could interact and be alert to signs that this may be happening. There are several good textbooks dealing with the uses and actions of individual medicines, including interactions. However, these will not be discussed here because at this stage of your career you are not expected to have a detailed knowledge of particular medicines, but rather an understanding of the key principles.

As nurses, we are concerned with how the body handles medicines (pharmacokinetics) so that we can see how this may be affected by age, genetics, or illness, and how the actions of medicines may conflict with one another or produce toxicity because their effects are additive. Equally, we need to look at occasions in which two medicines produce the same response by two different routes; such interactions can be beneficial to the patient and avoid having to give large doses of a single medicine because the same result can be achieved with smaller doses of two medicines, thereby reducing the risk of adverse effects.

You also need to understand what interactions there might be between different medicines and recognize when it may not be safe to administer a particular one. For example, you would question the prescribing of a monoamine oxidase inhibitor (MAOI) (medicines used to treat depression) to a patient with Parkinson's disease who was receiving levodopa, because MAOIs can trigger a hypertensive crisis when given with levodopa. Similarly, you would not want to administer digoxin to a patient with a pulse rate of less than 60 beats per minute because digoxin itself slows the heart (Sweetman, 2011). These are not necessarily things that you would be expected to know early in your nursing career, but they are learned with experience.

Now, you may already be feeling concerned about your knowledge of pharmacodynamics and pharmacokinetics. You are not alone and it is interesting to note that, in 2009, a survey of over 500 nurses from the Association for Nurse Prescribing database found that three-quarters of them felt they needed more education and training in the pharmacology of medicines (Lomas, 2009).

By the end of this chapter you should be feeling more confident about pharmacology. This in turn will enable you to better explain to your patients how drugs work and provide the necessary information to achieve concordance and keep patients safe. We will start by looking at how medicine enters the body and how this affects both the pharmacokinetics (how medicines are absorbed) and pharmacodynamics (how medicines work).

Box 3.2 Pharmacodynamics, pharmacokinetics, and pharmaceutics

Pharmacodynamics is how a medicine acts on the body.
Pharmacokinetics is how the body acts on the medicine.
Pharmaceutics is the preparation of a raw drug into a form in which it can be used to treat patients.

Basic pharmacokinetics

In order for a drug to act, sufficient quantities of the drug must reach the site of action, which will be an organ, tissue, or substance in the body, and remain there for sufficient time to produce their response. For a medicine taken internally (that is, not applied to a surface) the drug will go through four phases or steps:

- Absorption
- Distribution
- Metabolism
- Excretion.

That is, the drug must enter the body, move around the body to the site of action, and the body will dismantle the drug, and eject it. It is not necessary for each phase to end before the next one can start; as a result these four phases can overlap to some degree—but obviously the body cannot move what has not been absorbed.

It is also worth noting that pharmacokinetics depend upon the individual patient, in whom the efficiency of absorption, distribution, metabolism, and elimination may all vary. We will provide lots of examples along the way.

Absorption

Absorption will usually include the time taken for the drug to escape from the dosage form. The way in which a medicine is formulated and administered to the patient affects how quickly or slowly it is absorbed (Jambhekar and Breen, 2009). This can be vitally important in situations where patients are in a lot of pain or where a long lasting effect is desired.

Rate of absorption

Most ordinary tablets will have dissolved within an hour, but it is possible to vary the absorption time by changing the dosage form. For example, when a drug is injected intravenously, there is no absorption time because the drug has already reached the bloodstream and begun to circulate, so the drug goes directly to the distribution phase. There is no absorption phase in this case (Figure 3.1).

Once the medicine is in the circulation, the processes of metabolism and excretion do not differ, so the two curves have a similar shape, but because the

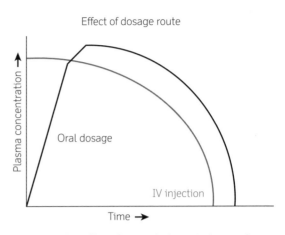

Figure 3.1 The effect of route of administration on drug concentrations.

intravenous injection does not have an **absorption step** the maximum concentration is reached immediately and the drug starts to work much faster. However, metabolism can start earlier too, so the duration of action (the length of time for which the drug works) is also shorter.

Liquids release their drugs more quickly than tablets, and soluble tablets dissolve more quickly than standard tablets. When we need a drug to act quickly, we may be able to formulate it in a quick-dissolving form. One example is rizatriptan, which is used for migraine, and can be prescribed in a thin tablet that dissolves very quickly on the patient's tongue.

Conversely, sometimes we want to slow down absorption, often because we want to extend the action of a drug. Slow release tablets can be used for this purpose. There are various ways to inhibit drug release, but for our purposes we may describe the two main methods. The ingredient can be wrapped in such a way that it is harder for the drug to escape, either by coating the whole tablet, or by enclosing the drug in little pellets within a capsule or tablet. You may have seen some flu or cold remedies that you can buy over the counter that consist of a capsule with little pellets inside to make their effect last longer. Alternatively, a matrix tablet can be used, which is made like a tiny sponge with small channels in it. The drug is at the centre and because the path to the outside is narrow and twisted, it takes time for the drug to escape. From the nursing point of view these matrix tablets pose a special challenge, because commonly the matrix itself is passed out of the body in the faeces and patients may think that this means that they did not receive any drug. You may need to explain that what is passed is just an empty shell.

As an added complication, it is possible to make tablets with both ordinary release and slow release layers bonded together like a sandwich. One leading brand of oxycodone tablet popular in palliative care is made like this. The ordinary layer releases the painkiller quickly, so the patient gets an early effect, but then the slow release layer releases a second batch of drug that means pain relief lasts for up to twelve hours. A tablet that only had the slow release layer would also last that long, but the patient would have to wait much longer for it to start acting.

It should also be noted that sometimes poor absorption of a medicine is good. The antibiotic vancomycin is used in some forms of colitis. It is usually poorly absorbed, which means that concentrations in the intestine remain high. However, in patients with severe inflammation of the intestine, absorption can be sufficiently high when large doses are given that toxicity results (Armstrong and Wilson, 1995).

Site of absorption

Quite often a medicine must be absorbed in a particular part of the gastrointestinal tract. For example, some would be destroyed by the high acidity of the stomach. This can be avoided by giving the tablet an acid-resistant coating that allows it to release its contents into the small intestine instead. These tablets used to be called enteric-coated, but the term **gastroresistant** is now preferred in official documents such as the *British National Formulary* (BNF). The antibiotic erythromycin is usually prescribed in gastroresistant tablets, but there are many other examples. For obvious reasons, a gastroresistant tablet must not be crushed or broken before administration, because that breaks the coating protecting the drug inside.

Although our skin seems very solid to us, it is possible to give some medicines through the skin in the form of transdermal patches. These slowly release the drug inside through the skin to which they are attached, and have the advantage that they can continue to do so for several days. Nicotine replacement patches for smokers are of this type, but the system is also used for painkillers and for some anti-angina drugs. Lately there has been great interest in adopting this method for a range of long-term conditions such as Parkinson's disease, because the patient's needs are relatively constant. Transdermal patches provide a very steady slow dribble of medication over a long time, which can give them a very long period of use, but also means that they take several hours to release enough medicine for the patient to feel an effect. For this reason the dosage can be difficult to adjust and they are rarely suitable for drugs where an immediate effect is needed.

One drug commonly given by transdermal patch is fentanyl, which is a strong painkiller often used in palliative care. A number of concerns have been raised recently about the use of fentanyl and similar patches and these will be explored in Exercise 3.1.

Clinical example

Fentanyl is an effective drug and has become particularly popular in care homes because the staff do not need to give repeated painkillers—the patch will last for 72 hours. The small transparent patch can be attached in an inaccessible part of the body reducing the chance that a confused patient will pull it off, and if patients have swallowing difficulties then a skin patch avoids having to give doses via a tube.

However, these same features also lead to the problems that have been observed.

1 The patch lasts for an average of 72 hours, but for some patients the patch lasts for a longer or shorter time.

2 The very fact that changes are infrequent increases the chance that staff will forget to change it unless

Exercise 3.1

Think for a moment about the kind of problems that might arise when a strong painkiller is given using a patch. List as many as you can think of.

there is a good system for recording the times when a change is due.

3 Sometimes staff fail to notice or cannot find a small transparent patch on the patient, especially if it has been deliberately placed somewhere inaccessible, with the result that the patient may be given another painkiller because their patch has not been noted. This can happen when a patient using a patch is admitted to hospital in an emergency and their notes are not available to the admissions team.

4 A potential problem is that absorption through the skin is dependent on temperature. If the patient is warm—and care homes can be very warm places—absorption will increase and the patient may overdose.

5 Fentanyl is effective and one way nurses know that it is working is that the patient reports fewer episodes of breakthrough pain—that is, acute pain that is not prevented by the fentanyl. There is a temptation to increase the fentanyl dose until the patient reports little or no breakthrough pain and then to maintain that dose, but unless the dose is reduced from time to time we have no way of knowing if it is still needed. If the dose is not needed, then we are giving our patients a powerful drug with a real risk of harming their health without gaining any additional benefit from it, which must be poor practice.

The MHRA publication *Fentanyl patches: serious and fatal overdose from dosing errors, accidental exposure, and inappropriate use* (2008) describes these and other problems. See also Larsen et al (2003), where individual variation is described.

How do drugs enter tissues?

The most common method by which drugs move out of the circulation and into cells is by simple diffusion (see Figure 3.2). The drug molecules cross the semi-permeable membranes surrounding the cells because the concentration of drug inside the cell is less than that outside. This process does not use energy.

The molecules of drug in the blood stream will pass into the adjoining cell because the concentration of

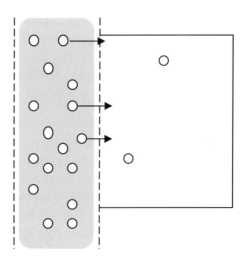

Figure 3.2 Simple diffusion.

drug there is lower. This would not be possible if the cell membrane was solid.

However, there are other mechanisms that may be involved. In facilitated diffusion (see Figures 3.3a and b) there are carrier molecules that assist the drug to pass, either by piggybacking the drug to the carrier or because the carrier attaches to the membrane and causes channels to open through which the drug can pass.

The body has active transport mechanisms that use energy to transport natural chemicals against a concentration gradient. This is commonly seen when the body recycles chemicals for reuse later, but the same mechanisms can sometimes be used to help the body absorb medicines. For example, some synthetic versions of vitamins are absorbed using the active transport mechanisms that would normally trap natural dietary vitamins. Just for completeness we should note that active transport may also work to remove substances from cells. One mechanism by which bacteria develop resistance to antibiotics may be by using active transport mechanisms to push the drug out of their cells (Dever, 2000; Wu et al, 2005). Energy is needed because the substance is actively transported against the gradient, just as you need energy to push a ball uphill.

Finally, a very small number of drugs are absorbed by pinocytosis in which droplets of the liquid drug are engulfed by the cell (see Figure 3.4a and b). The

(a)

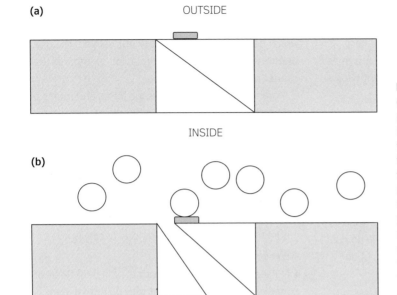

OUTSIDE

INSIDE

(b)

Figure 3.3 Facilitated diffusion.
(a) The membrane of this cell contains a protein molecule (drawn in white), which bridges the membrane so that one side is inside the cell and the other face is outside the cell. The outside surface has a receptor or target for the molecule that is going to pass.
(b) When the molecule combines with the receptor, it causes a change in the protein's shape such that a channel is made through to the inside of the cell. The molecule is then able to pass through to the interior by ordinary diffusion because the concentration there is lower. Again, no energy is needed to allow this.

(a)

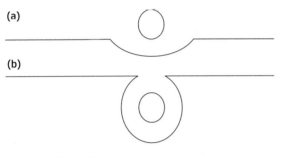

(b)

Figure 3.4 Pinocytosis.
(a) The membrane develops a bowl into which the molecule to be trapped arrives. The bowl deepens until it encloses the molecule.
(b) The two sides meet and close over, then the bubble pops at the bottom to let the molecule escape into the interior of the cell.

membrane of the cell forms a pocket in which the liquid sits, and then the arms of the cell close around it to trap the liquid. The membrane breaks and reforms so that the liquid is now inside the reformed cell.

An example of a medicine absorbed in this way is cyanocobalamin (vitamin B_{12}), which forms a complex with intrinsic factor in the duodenum and then passes through the mucosa of the terminal ileum by pinocytosis. (Dharmarajan et al, 2003).

Exercise 3.2

Make a list of the factors that you think might affect the absorption of drugs given orally. Then do the same for drugs applied to the skin.

Factors that affect the absorption of oral drugs

A large number of factors affect absorption of oral drugs. These include:

- The quality of the mucosa lining the gastrointestinal tract. Patients such as those with coeliac disease may have difficulty in absorbing drugs because their mucosa is flattened.
- The presence of stomach contents such as food reduces absorption, and there may also be interactions with the food that reduce the availability of drug. For example, the antibiotic tetracycline binds to the calcium in milk making it harder to absorb.
- Absorption depends to some extent on the time for which the drug is in contact with the mucosa, so if the patient has a hyperactive or unusually slow gut, absorption may change. Similarly, if the blood flow is

slow, then the concentration gradient across the blood vessel membrane will decrease, slowing absorption.

- The degree of acidity of the stomach may affect absorption too, and for those drugs where enzymes assist absorption, changes in enzyme quantity or quality will have an effect.

Similar factors control absorption through skin:

- By mixing the drug in either a cream base (which is largely water) or an ointment base (which is largely oil or fat) we can change the extent to which the drug either lies on or penetrates the skin.

- Absorption is quickest and more complete where the skin is thin, which is one reason why we do not commonly absorb much through the soles of our feet.

- Dry, cool skin absorbs less than warm, moist skin, so temperature and hydration are important, and the blood flow carrying the absorbed drug away is also important; in the elderly and newborn babies, blood flow may be poor and absorption is reduced.

Sometimes we do not want to promote absorption. Steroid creams are intended to work at or near the skin surface and we want absorption kept to a minimum.

When a drug is injected intravenously, 100% of the dose reaches the patient's circulation. When any other route is used, it is common to find that a proportion is lost on the way. It fails to leave the dosage form, or is destroyed before it is absorbed, and the absorption process is not perfectly efficient. After it is absorbed, the first pass mechanism (described later) may prevent the medicine reaching the systemic circulation.

As a result, we may find that only 70–80% of a dose is received by the body. This is called the **fractional bioavailability**, or sometimes just the bioavailability. Note that this is not constant for a drug, because it depends on the form in which it is given. For example, the anti-asthma drug salbutamol has higher bioavailability from syrup than from tablets. The availability from an aerosol inhaler is surprisingly small, but because the proportion absorbed all reaches the airways, it will produce better results than a tablet, which has better bioavailability but delivers the drug to the whole body, including a lot of organs that cannot use it.

More information about dosage forms and routes of administration can be found in Chapter 4.

Review of absorption

- The absorption time includes the time taken for the drug to escape from the dosage form.

- The formulation of medicine and route of administration affects how quickly or slowly it is absorbed.

- Nurses should be familiar with the different types of medication available so that they do not interfere with the characteristics of a special formulation by using it wrongly, for example, crushing the coating of a slow release tablet.

- Nurses can anticipate the factors that can affect the absorption of drugs whether given orally, applied to the skin, or administered by another route.

- By understanding the bioavailability of a medication, nurses can suggest various formulations to maximize benefits to their patients and explain to patients what to expect.

Distribution

You may be very familiar with the saying that oil and water do not mix. That is generally true of the internal environment of the human body too. You will learn in your physiology studies that body fluids usually consist largely of water, while the cells of the body are enclosed in membranes made of lipids, which are fats. Water-soluble drugs will concentrate in body fluids, while lipid-soluble drugs will collect in body fat. The terms we commonly use are **hydrophilic** (water-loving) and **lipophilic** (fat-loving).

A number of factors affect the distribution of drugs within the body. They can be divided into two main

Table 3.1 Factors affecting drug distribution.

Properties of the drug	Properties of the patient
Lipid solubility	Age
Affinity for plasma or tissue proteins	Ethnic origin
Ability to cross blood–brain barrier	Body composition
Size of the molecules	General state of health

groups—those that are properties of the drug, and those which are properties of the patient. See Table 3.1.

To some extent these may be inter-related. Ethnic origin, for example, affects body composition, and molecular size influences the ability to cross the blood–brain barrier (Jambhekar and Breen, 2009).

The blood–brain barrier

Blood is transported to the brain as to any other organ, but the brain itself is mainly supplied by cerebrospinal fluid. This receives substances such as glucose from the blood, but the two liquids are kept apart by a layer of cells lining the capillaries that have tight junctions; that is, they do not contain the small gaps through which substances can usually enter and leave capillaries. This protects the brain from a range of noxious chemicals that might be found in the blood.

Comparatively few drugs can cross this barrier, but those that can tend to have very small molecules that are lipophilic. Hydrophilic molecules are retained in the blood.

The effects of penetration of the blood–brain barrier can sometimes be seen within a group of drugs. For example, the beta-blocker propranolol is sometimes used in the treatment of migraine, whilst some other beta-blockers such as atenolol are not useful. This is because propranolol is lipophilic and crosses the blood–brain barrier more easily than other beta-blockers, but this also carries a penalty, because patients may complain of disturbed sleep and vivid nightmares with propranolol. This happens precisely because it can enter the brain, and is very unusual with other drugs in the group. With atenolol, for example, the concentration of drug in the brain can be

as low as one tenth of that in the general circulation because it cannot pass the blood–brain barrier so easily (Cruickshank et al, 1980).

The importance of protein binding

For many drugs, a proportion of each dose attaches temporarily to proteins in the blood, and is therefore not free to act—it is described as 'bound'.

In the next section we will explain metabolism fully, but for now, it can be defined as the mechanism by which the body dismantles medicines. A drug enters the general circulation as it is absorbed, and leaves it as it is metabolized. Drug molecules that are bound are generally protected from metabolism, but unbound drug molecules can be metabolized. The body tries to maintain a balance or equilibrium between bound and unbound drug, so the proportion of the drug that is bound does not change. As a drug leaves the general circulation through metabolism, some of the bound drug will become free to maintain the same proportions of free to bound drug, until eventually the bound drug is released. This extends the duration of action of the drug, because the proteins act as a reservoir of drug, and the bound drug is generally protected from the enzymes that would destroy it if it were free (Figure 3.5).

If all the drug were free, metabolism would be much quicker. If, in our example, it takes the enzymes 30 minutes to destroy the drug molecule, then potentially if there were no protein binding the whole dose could be destroyed in that time. However, because bound drug is preserved from attack, after half an hour only a third of the drug can be destroyed. It will take over two hours (at least four cycles of destruction and unbinding) to remove the drug in this example.

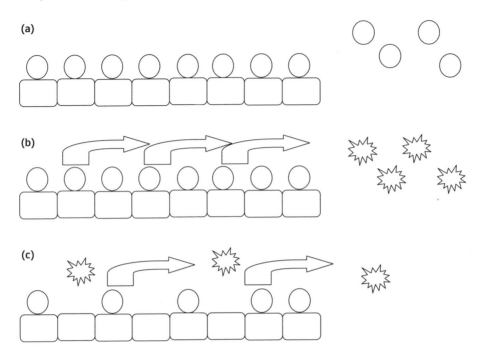

Figure 3.5 Protein binding.
(a) In this (highly simplified) example, eight molecules of drug are bound to a protein, while four are free in the circulation, so one-third of the drug is unbound.
(b) Enzymes acting on the free drug destroy it. To maintain the balance of free to bound drug, some of the bound drug has to become unbound.
(c) As more of the free drug is metabolized, the reservoir of bound drug becomes depleted until there may be no bound drug left.

This binding is not permanent; the drug separates and rebinds many times, but at any given moment a snapshot would reveal a consistent fraction of drug to be bound. For most drugs, the percentage that will be bound is predictable, at least for a population, though with less certainty for any individual person. Warfarin, for example, is usually about 97% bound. That means that only 3% of a dose of warfarin is active at any given time (Ashraful Alam et al, 2008).

This figure immediately explains the importance of protein binding. If a patient receiving warfarin is simultaneously given another drug that binds to plasma proteins, one of the drugs may not be able to bind as usual because a given amount of blood only has a limited number of binding sites, and only one drug can bind to any particular site at a time. Over three-quarters of a dose of aspirin is usually protein-bound, but if a patient is given aspirin and warfarin

at the same time, it is likely that some of the warfarin will be displaced from the protein. As a result the percentage that is bound might drop from 97% to 96%. This may seem unimportant, but remember that the blood-thinning effect of warfarin that we see is being produced by just 3% of the dose, the portion that is free. If the bound fraction drops to 96%, then the free portion increases from 3% to 4%. That means that the amount of free warfarin increases by one-third, which may increase the risk of haemorrhage in some patients.

The proteins that drugs bind to are typically serum albumin and globulins. Protein binding is a significant factor when a drug binds readily to those proteins, particularly if another protein-binding drug is also given. However, patients can also experience difficulty if the binding capacity of their blood changes for other reasons.

Kidney and liver disease can change the binding of drugs to protein because of a decrease in protein (e.g. decreased albumin in nephrotic syndrome or liver disease) or as a result of competition for protein binding by substances produced in the body (e.g. uraemia in kidney disease or hyperbilirubinaemia in liver disease).

Exercise 3.3

This table shows a list of drugs and the typical percentage of a dose of these drugs that is protein bound. Even if you know very little about the drugs, you should be able to guess which of them might pose problems when given with warfarin.

Carbamazepine	75% bound
Digoxin	25% bound
Lithium	0% bound
Phenobarbital	30% bound
Phenytoin	90% bound
Sodium valproate	90% bound

The drugs we would be concerned about are carbamazepine, phenytoin, and sodium valproate. They are all highly protein bound and there may be competition for protein binding sites between any of these drugs and warfarin, which will push warfarin into the blood and increase the amount of free warfarin. The clinical importance is that these medicines are all used in epilepsy, where avoiding changes in plasma concentration of drugs can be extremely important.

Review of distribution

- Distribution describes the way in which the drug passes from the site of absorption to the site of action and the rest of the body.
- The pattern of distribution is affected by the differing solubilities of drugs, some of which are more lipid-soluble while others are more water-soluble.
- Distribution is inhibited by protein binding, which therefore creates a reservoir of drug that can be used over a longer period of time.

Metabolism

Later in this chapter we will discuss how drugs act at their target sites, but for the moment let us think of the action of a drug as rather like a finger pressing a doorbell. When the drug reaches its target organ it makes contact and produces a result, just as a finger pressing on a bell produces a noise.

It would be very awkward if the finger never left the bell again. The bell would not be free for other fingers, and the continuing noise would be irritating and would serve no purpose, because you would already have answered the door. In the same way, if a drug reached an organ and produced an effect, and then continued to produce it indefinitely, it would be very inconvenient. A drug that causes your heart to slow might be useful, but not if makes it beat slower and slower without end. We therefore need a way of breaking the connection between a drug and its target, and the simplest way is to destroy the drug.

Moreover, so far as the body is concerned a drug is usually a foreign substance. The body has systems designed to remove foreign chemicals in case they are toxic. These systems depend on enzymes that together make a toolkit of different ways to dismantle or change a foreign chemical and make it harmless.

The collection of chemical reactions that happen within us to maintain life is called metabolism, from a Greek word meaning 'to change'. Metabolism takes place throughout the body and you will often come across the term to describe how food is converted into energy. In pharmacology, the metabolism that takes place in the liver is particularly important, and therefore we will describe processes in the liver as the typical example (but do not forget that metabolism happens elsewhere too—in the epithelium of the intestinal tract, the lungs, kidneys and skin, for example).

Drugs are usually metabolized in two phases. In the first phase of metabolism, enzymes work on the drug to make it more chemically reactive or more water-soluble. In the second phase, the activated drug is attached to another carrier molecule such as glucuronic acid to make it easier to excrete, either in the urine or in the faeces. Those excreted in urine are normally returned to the circulation and then extracted by the kidneys. Some will conjugate with bile acids and pass into the intestine and hence to the faeces.

Let us see an example of metabolism in action. Figure 3.6a shows the chemical structure of the painkiller oxycodone.

The thick black lines are an attempt to draw a three-dimensional shape on a flat page. For our purposes the exact structure is unimportant. Imagine that the three hexagons form a flat plate on the surface of the page. The nitrogen atom N is in a handle that pokes out of the page towards us. At the far end there is a little tail including an oxygen atom O. During the first phase of metabolism, enzymes attack the bonds to these methyl groups to snip them off. They may snip off the N-methyl group first (marked with an asterisk in Figure 3.6), or the O-methyl group first (marked with a cross in the diagram), so they can produce two 'daughter' molecules (Figure 3.6b and c).

In time, both methyl groups may be removed. The result is a much more reactive molecule that readily binds to other water-soluble molecules like glucuronates. The resulting complex is more easily excreted than the original drug. These glucuronates, which are much bigger molecules, attach where the methyl group has been cut off. This process of attaching the metabolized drug onto a carrier is called **conjugation**. Because the combination of a large carrier molecule and a smaller molecule looks rather like an adult giving a child a piggy-back, it is sometimes described as 'piggy-backing'. The conjugated drug is much more soluble in water and therefore less likely to enter cells, but more likely to pass into the urine at the kidney. In this way the body rids itself of any oxycodone that we take. For a drug to be useful, it must be able to act before the body destroys it. This may seem obvious, but it explains why we may have to give drugs in a particular way.

First pass metabolism

The enzymes that destroy drugs are present in large quantities in the liver. Ideally, therefore, we would give our drug the best chance of producing its effect if we could keep it away from the liver. Unfortunately, this is not easy, because almost all of our blood passes through the liver each minute, and there is a vein that takes absorbed material from the stomach directly to the liver—the hepatic portal vein. If the liver enzymes are efficient in destroying the drug, it may therefore be almost useless.

However, some parts of the circulation are more remote from the liver, and drugs absorbed there have a chance to act before being transported to the liver. One such site is the lining of the mouth. The anti-angina drug glyceryl trinitrate is commonly given as either a spray or tiny tablets which are placed under the tongue. The drug is quickly absorbed and speedily eases the chest pain that angina produces. If the patient swallows their tablet, it will be ineffective, because the liver enzymes will destroy the active ingredient before it has had a chance to act.

This quick destruction of the drug is called the first pass effect; that is, the drug is destroyed because it first passes through the liver. Suppositories may also avoid the first pass effect, because the blood supply for the lower two-thirds of the rectum allows a drug to be absorbed without passage through the liver first.

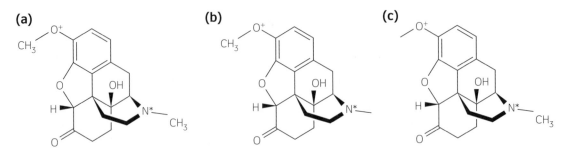

Figure 3.6 (a) The chemical structure of oxycodone, (b) and (c) The chemical structure of the two 'daughter' molecules which may be produced.

Prodrugs

Most drugs enter the body in an inactive state and rely on metabolism to make them active. These are called prodrugs. The antihypertensive drug enalapril is a good example of a prodrug. Its makers originally produced a drug called enalaprilat. This was effective, but its absorption was very poor, so it could only be used as an injection. To overcome this, the researchers combined enalaprilat with alcohol to make the drug enalapril which is much more readily absorbed from a tablet. Enalapril is not an active drug, but within the body enalapril is acted upon by enzymes to give the original enalaprilat, which is active (MacFadyen et al, 1993).

Sometimes we do not realize that a drug is a prodrug. This was the case with the steroid drug prednisone, which is converted in the body to prednisolone. When this was discovered, it became common to give prednisolone directly to patients because there is no advantage in using prednisone and the time taken by the body to convert it to prednisolone delays treatment slightly so prednisone is not seen in the United Kingdom today. However, it is still prescribed in some countries in place of prednisolone, possibly due to prescribers' familiarity with it.

Cytochrome enzymes

There are a large number of enzymes that are involved in the metabolism of drugs in the body, but the most common group are the cytochrome enzymes. They are sometimes known as cytochrome P450 enzymes. The cyto- part of their name indicates that they are found inside cells, and the –chrome suffix is related to their ability to absorb light, particularly at a wavelength of 450 nanometres. There is an explanation of the naming of cytochromes and a fuller explanation of light absorption at: **http://www.anaesthetist.com/physiol/basics/metabol/cyp/Findex.htm**.

These enzymes are involved in oxidation reactions—that is, they add oxygen to molecules to make them more reactive. Cytochrome enzymes are therefore very important for the first phase of metabolism.

There are over 11 000 different cytochrome enzymes found throughout our bodies but particularly in the liver. The particular enzymes that we each have are determined genetically. While we all have broadly similar collections of cytochrome enzymes, they will differ according to the genes our parents gave us, with close relatives being more likely to have similar enzymes. Conversely, some populations or ethnic groups may lack a particular enzyme. A number of Asian people are lacking an enzyme that plays a key role in metabolizing the anti-cholesterol drug rosuvastatin, so for people from these ethnic groups it is customary to halve the dose, because they find it harder to remove the drug and hence it could accumulate in their bodies if they were given full doses (Liao, 2007).

Cytochrome enzymes are named according to a system. Their name usually begins with CYP. It is then followed by a numeral describing its family, then a letter to describe its sub-family, and finally another number (which may have more than one digit) to describe the particular form present. For example, the enzyme CYP2C9 is very important in the metabolism of warfarin. The closely-related enzyme CYP2C19—pronounced to end with 'nineteen'—is involved in metabolizing diazepam and omeprazole. We know that they must be closely related because they share the family number 2 and the sub-family letter C. We can regard these as a bit like surnames, whereas the last number is rather like our first names.

Polymorphism

Enzymes are large and complex proteins built from amino-acids. Within their structures they may incorporate some differences without losing their identity. For example, they may have slightly different amino-acids in particular places. Alternatively, sequences of genes may have been repeated in a person's DNA which causes repetitions in the proteins produced. Having multiple copies of a single enzyme is called polymorphism, from Greek words meaning 'many bodies'.

These changes in structure may be unimportant, but in some cases they may make a difference to the efficiency of the enzyme or the extent to which it is able to fulfil its role. Repetitions may also mean that a person has a much larger quantity of an enzyme than the average.

CYP2C19 is an example of genetic polymorphism; that is, there are a large number of molecules that are all variations of CYP2C19, sometimes with amino-acids swapped over or missing. As a result, some versions of CYP2C19 are not very active. Around 20% of Asian patients have a type of CYP2C19 that is not effective, as a result of which they are called slow metabolizers (Goldstein et al, 1997). When they are given drugs metabolized by CYP2C19 the dose may have to be reduced to prevent its accumulation in their bodies. Since 80% of Asian patients do not have this enzyme variant, the prescriber will usually give the normal dose of drugs that might be effective, but may ask the nurses to watch for signs of side effects that suggest that the drug level is building up, in which event the dose will have to be reduced.

Enzyme induction and inhibition

These enzymes can be induced (made more active or increased in amount) or inhibited (made less active) by other drugs or dietary constituents. For example, the enzyme CYP1A2 is inhibited by the antibiotic ciprofloxacin, caffeine, and by some natural

Box 3.3 Clopidogrel

Clopidogrel is a medicine used to prevent blood clotting. It is a prodrug that is converted by CYP2C19 to the active form. In patients who are slow metabolizers—that is, they have a less active variant of CYP2C19—the amount of active drug that they produce is much reduced, and clopidogrel may not give them the protection that they need. In the United States, the Food and Drug Administration has instructed manufacturers to include a warning to prescribers in their literature to remind them that the drug can be less effective in people who cannot metabolize the drug to convert it to its active form. The safety notice can be found at: **http://www.fda.gov/Drugs/DrugSafety/ PostmarketDrugSafetyInformationforPatientsand Providers/ucm203888.htm**.

chemicals found in Seville oranges or grapefruit juice and induced by nicotine—there are tables of enzyme inducers and inhibitors at: **http://www. fda.gov/Drugs/DevelopmentApprovalProcess/ DevelopmentResources/DrugInteractionsLabeling/ ucm093664.htm**.

If the enzyme is inhibited, it will not destroy the drugs it is expected to work upon, so they will build up in the body and may cause adverse effects. This explains why patients given some drugs such as the antihypertensive drug felodipine are told not to drink grapefruit juice.

Those substances that cause enzyme induction tend to do so for many cytochrome enzymes. Equally, those that inhibit are not selective and do so for most cytochrome enzymes. There is often a subtle difference between these two groups. Inhibitors compete for the enzyme with the substances the enzyme would normally attack. Since at least part of the capacity of the enzyme is taken up with dealing with the inhibitor, the activity of the enzyme is reduced. For this reason, the inhibition starts immediately the inhibitor is present and is related to the dose of the inhibitor.

Inducers, however, commonly cause an increase in the amount of enzyme. There is therefore a delay before induction takes place while new enzyme is made, and there may not be a direct relationship between the quantity of inducer and the effect seen.

There are many enzyme inducers, but amongst the most common are phenobarbital, phenytoin, carbamazepine, nicotine, and rifampicin. The first three of these may all be given in epilepsy. Since inducers increase the metabolic activity of the cytochrome enzymes, those enzymes work harder and destroy other drugs more quickly, so it can be very challenging to find the right dose of other treatments for patients with epilepsy. Even when a dose appears to be correct, induction of enzymes by antiepileptic drugs may promote the other drug's destruction and may mean that later the dose will be insufficient.

There are fewer enzyme inhibitors, but they include cimetidine, monoamine oxidase inhibitors, quinolone antibiotics (such as ciprofloxacin) and macrolide antibiotics such as erythromycin and clarithromycin.

You will not be expected to have a comprehensive knowledge of enzyme inducers and inhibitors as an undergraduate nurse. It is sufficient to know that they exist, to be able to give one or two examples, and to understand the key effect of each group.

Enzyme inducers increase enzyme activity or the amount of enzyme, so other drugs are destroyed more quickly, which lowers the levels of those drugs in the blood.

Enzyme inhibitors reduce enzyme activity, so other drugs are destroyed more slowly, allowing the blood levels of those drugs to rise as if the patient had been given a bigger dose.

This may seem to be only of academic interest, but a simple example may serve to show that an alert nurse can help their patients considerably.

Clinical example

You will have noticed that nicotine was included in the list of enzyme inducers. People who smoke may metabolize drugs more quickly as a result, so if we need to keep their blood levels high we may have to increase their dose. Many smokers are prone to breathing difficulties, and as a result they may be prescribed drugs of the theophylline family. These open the airways to aid breathing, but they have the side-effect of causing nausea at higher doses and can leave patients feeling very queasy (BNF, 2012).

Since smoking induces cytochrome enzymes, the prescriber may have to increase the dose of theophylline to the point where it would normally cause nausea, except that the induced enzymes metabolize it quickly. If the patient then agrees to stop smoking, their nicotine levels will slowly fall, and the enzyme induction will be reversed. As a result, their metabolism of theophylline will slow down, and the levels of theophylline in the patient's blood will start to rise—and remember that their dose may well have been high to begin with. This can leave the patient feeling very ill, and since the only change that they have brought about is to stop smoking, they may think that quitting has made them ill, which makes it harder to persuade them to persevere. An alert nurse could suggest to the patient that they speak to their doctor about slowly reducing their theophylline dose after they have stopped smoking, which will reduce the risk of nausea.

If you have understood enzyme inhibition and induction, the example just given should make sense to you. If it does not, you may want to review this section again.

Review of metabolism

- Substances entering the body are metabolized to make them easier to remove. Metabolism uses enzymes, and each person's enzymes are determined by their genetics.

- As a result, some people lack the enzymes needed to destroy particular drugs, or have less efficient versions of those enzymes.

- In the first stage of metabolism, these enzymes chemically alter the drug to make it more ready to react chemically with other substances in the body.

- In the second stage of metabolism, the altered drug is attached to a molecule (usually more water-soluble) to aid excretion.

- This process of attachment is called conjugation.

Excretion

Most drugs are excreted in either urine or faeces, or both, with the kidneys being the major route of excretion for many. However, it is important to note that there are other ways that drugs or their metabolites can be expelled from the body.

Iron is primarily excreted in faeces. The antiepileptic drugs phenytoin and sodium valproate are excreted in saliva. This is very convenient, because adjustment of doses to maintain desired blood levels is very important, but it is distressing to children to take repeated samples of blood to check their dosage. However, because these drugs are excreted in saliva, a sample of saliva can be tested because the level there is related in a known way to the blood level. If we know one, we can work out the other.

Some drugs are excreted in breast milk. (Breast milk may also contain drugs which have not yet been metabolized.) There are two reasons to be wary of drugs in breast milk.

Obviously these drugs could damage the infant, which is a concern with some sleeping tablets. A relatively small dose for the mother may pass to the infant as a dose that they cannot metabolize and which therefore puts them at risk. Although such examples are known, generally prescribers are very careful about prescribing for breast-feeding mothers and it is unusual to find babies being put at risk in this way. Even when these drugs must be used, it is normal to persuade the mother to stop breast-feeding until the course of treatment is over. For example, a number of anti-cancer drugs pass into breast milk and may cause damage to the infant. If a mother has cancer, she cannot wait for treatment until her baby is no longer feeding, and she will be counselled to give her baby formula milk so that the treatment can commence.

A more likely problem is that an ingredient in a medicine may affect the milk so that the baby will not feed properly. Some mothers will report that if they have to take cough medicines their babies dislike their milk. A striking example of a medicine affecting breast milk is that of the antiseptic povidone-iodine, which may concentrate in breast milk and turn it orange. Even at levels that do not cause the baby harm, povidone-iodine may discourage proper feeding.

Key pharmacokinetic concepts

Half-life

Figure 3.7 shows the typical course of the concentration of a drug in the blood stream after an oral dose. One key concept remains to be discussed, the half-life; this is the time it takes for the level of drug in the plasma to drop by half. In the example in the figure, peak concentration is reached 2.5 hours after the medicine is taken. If you follow the line across from the 50% concentration mark, you can see that this will be reached after 6.5 hours, so the half-life in this case is 4 hours. If you then see when the concentration will be halved again, it is the point at which the concentration is reduced to 25%, at 10.5 hours.

For most drugs the half-life is relatively constant, so if the initial concentration is 100%, after one half-life it has dropped to 50%, after two half-lives to 25%, and so on. After five half-lives it is a little over 3%, and we

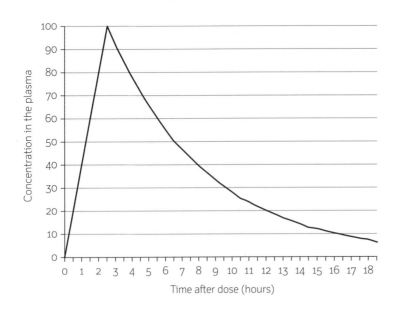

Figure 3.7 Changes in the plasma concentration of a drug following an oral dose.

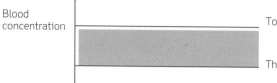

Figure 3.8 The therapeutic window. In this diagram the shaded area represents the therapeutic window.

normally regard five half-lives as the time a drug takes to clear the body after the last dose was taken. The half-life is usually denoted by $t_{1/2}$.

It is the half-life which determines the interval between doses. If the half-life is short, we will need to give doses more often than if it is long. For example, the antibiotic ampicillin has a half-life of a little over an hour. As a result, within six hours almost all the dose will have left the body and therefore we must give it at least four times a day. On the other hand, digoxin, which is given to control irregular heart rhythms and improve the contractility of the heart, has a half-life of about 36 hours. We commonly give it once a day, but in fact it can be given every other day because it is only slowly removed from the body.

The therapeutic window

This is an important concept, at least for drugs taken internally. A drug will not act until the concentration in the blood reaches an adequate level. This is called the **therapeutic level** (see Figure 3.8). If concentrations in the blood continue to increase the patient may begin to experience adverse effects, and the level at which this starts is called the **toxic level**. The range between the therapeutic and toxic levels is called the therapeutic window. The aim of treatment is to keep the drug level in the patient within this therapeutic window so that the patient gains the benefits of the drug without the side effects.

Unfortunately for some drugs the therapeutic window is very narrow. An example is the anti-asthma drug theophylline. For some patients the toxic level is actually lower than the therapeutic level, so they experience adverse effects before they derive any benefit.

Pharmacogenetics

As we shall see, pharmacodynamics of drugs barely differ between patients. If a hundred people are given a drug that lowers blood pressure, the degree of response may differ between them, but the type of response will not. It would be a surprise if it caused a rise in blood pressure in some of them.

This is not true of pharmacokinetics. Pharmacokinetics depend upon the individual patient, in whom the efficiency of absorption, distribution, metabolism, and elimination may all vary. Tables of pharmacokinetic values such as half-life and protein binding fraction are averages, but there will be wide variation around that average. For example, the half-life of the heart drug amiodarone is quoted as about 58 days, but it can vary from 15 to 142 days.

One key reason for this is the genetic basis for enzyme production and activity. Some of us produce fewer enzymes, are missing particular enzymes, or produce enzymes that are less effective than similar enzymes in other people. This basic fact has led to the development of a field of study called pharmacogenetics, which is the study of genetic variation that gives rise to differing responses to drugs.

An early example arose with the muscle relaxant suxamethonium, which was used during some operations to paralyse the patient. For the great majority of patients the paralysis was easily reversed once the drug was stopped, but for about 1 in 3500 patients the paralysis continued for a long time and was occasionally fatal. This was discovered to be due to a variation in an enzyme that we use to metabolize suxamethonium. These patients either did not possess this enzyme or had a version of it which was not very effective, with the result that they were unable to clear the suxamethonium from their body in the expected time.

Another example is that of codeine. Codeine is actually not a very powerful painkiller. Its effect is due to the fact that about 10% of the dose is converted to morphine in the liver by the enzyme CYP2D6. About 8–10% of the white population is believed to have a version of this enzyme which is inefficient and as result they do not make morphine. For them, codeine is a very poor painkiller (Ingelman-Sundberg, 2005). Unfortunately, sometimes prescribers interpret this poor response as evidence that they have not given enough, and therefore increase the dose. The patient can gain no benefit but will be exposed to a higher risk of adverse effects.

Normally about 80% of the codeine dose is metabolized by another liver enzyme, CYP3A4, to make norcodeine, which is conjugated and excreted. However, in patients who have low CYP3A4 levels, or who are receiving drugs like the antibiotic clarithromycin which inhibit CYP3A4, the slowing of this pathway allows more drug to be converted by CYP2D6. This may lead to morphine-induced side effects.

Conversely, some patients may have enzymes that are more efficient than the average. There is a case report (Gasche et al, 2004) describing a patient who had three types of CYP2D6, with the result that he was able to convert codeine to morphine very efficiently. As a result, even small doses of codeine cough medicine could produce life-threatening morphine side effects.

Review of pharmacogenetics

- Genetic differences lead to great variation in the way in which individuals are able to benefit from their medicines, and in the risks that they face from them.
- Enzymes play a key role in the metabolism of drugs and these tend to be affected by genetics in that some people have low levels or lack certain enzymes.
- Pharmacogenetics, which is the study of genetic variation that gives rise to differing responses to drugs, is likely to be studied more widely in the future.

Pharmacodynamics

Pharmacodynamics studies the effects of drugs at their sites of action. A drug's pharmacodynamics are predictable and do not vary in type—though they may in degree—between individuals. That is, a drug does the same thing to all of us. For example, insulin lowers blood sugar whenever it is given. It does not cause increases in blood sugar in some people.

It is beyond the scope of an introductory text like this to describe all the ways in which drugs can act. This chapter looks at four.

1 By attaching to receptors
2 By blocking the action of specific enzymes
3 By inhibiting cell transport mechanisms
4 By acting on invading organisms.

Drugs which act by attaching to receptors

Many drugs work by attaching themselves to a target which we call a **receptor**. Receptors differ in their structure, but they are generally proteins. When a drug reaches a matching receptor, it will trigger some sort of response there.

Earlier we used the analogy of a finger touching a doorbell, which makes the bell ring. The analogy is not exact, because any finger will work any bell—it would be a poor doorbell if some people's fingers did not make it chime. Indeed, a pointed stick will make it ring, as would a carrot, a magic wand, or a well-aimed pebble. The doorbell lacks specificity; its action is not specific to a particular stimulus.

Our receptors are much more selective. Their construction is quite complex, but we can gain a good understanding of their working by using a simple model.

The lock and key hypothesis

A key has to fit its lock, or it will not open the door. There is a physical relationship between them that enables them to do their job.

We can picture the relationship between a drug and its receptor as very similar to that between a key and

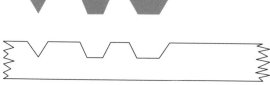

Figure 3.9 Recognition sites.

its lock. If the drug fits the receptor, it may be able to trigger the expected response. The fit does not have to be precise provided that it contains the right chemical groups in the right places.

In Figure 3.9 the drug molecule, shown in grey, has the right shape to fit the receptor, shown in white. So long as the three protruding groups are the right size and shape, and are the right distance apart, the rest of the drug molecule's structure is unimportant. It is the recognition groups that determine the fit.

Receptors do not exist to receive drug molecules. They are there to accept natural chemicals that are needed for the functioning of the organ where the receptor sits. For example, oxytocin stimulates labour by causing the uterine smooth muscle to contract, because its receptors are to be found there.

The natural chemical noradrenaline has the structure shown in Figure 3.10a, with the ball signifying an amine (-NH$_2$) group. The drug salbutamol, shown in Figure 3.10b, which mimics noradrenaline's actions on the airways, has the same shape except that the ball in this case consists of a much larger group where one of the hydrogen atoms of the NH$_2$ group has been replaced by a clump of 4 carbon atoms.

This change means that salbutamol is very effective in acting on the airways, but it does not have the cardiac side effects that noradrenaline has. From this we

deduce two things: the airways' β$_2$ receptors must be bound by parts of the molecule that do not involve the ball group at the end, because both noradrenaline and salbutamol will bind there; but the cardiac receptors must bind at the ball end because the larger group on salbutamol will not bind well. By manipulating molecules and seeing what effect the changes have on receptor binding, we can work out what the binding groups must be and where they have to be positioned.

For example, the drug terbutaline has very similar actions to salbutamol though its structure differs. The two groups attaching to the left of the ring as seen in Figure 3.10a and b are not side-by-side, as in salbutamol and noradrenaline, but have a larger gap between them. This suggests that at least one of those groups cannot be involved in binding to the receptor, or it would be in the wrong place.

The points on the receptor where the drug attaches are called **recognition sites**. When the correct bindings take place, the drug can trigger a response. Such a drug is called an **agonist**, which comes from a Greek word meaning to act—the drug acts at the receptor.

Receptor blockers and antagonists

Another possibility is that a drug can attach at some recognition sites, but not be sufficiently well attached to trigger a response. However, by attaching at all, it prevents the natural chemical or another drug from occupying the receptor. It can therefore block their action, in the same way that sometimes a key will fit in a lock but not be able to turn. To understand this, see the simplified example in Figure 3.11.

In this example, the receptor has three recognition sites, labelled A, B and C. An agonist would have to occupy all three sites in order to produce an effect. However, the shape above the receptor represents a drug that will fit sites A and B, but not C. As a result, other chemicals will not be able to bind at A or B, so they will be blocked. In this particular case, the drug physically blocks access to C too, without being able to attach there, but a molecule that was cut short at the dotted line would still block the receptor. These blockers are called **antagonists** (think of them as 'anti-agonists'). The drug group β-blockers (or beta-blockers) block

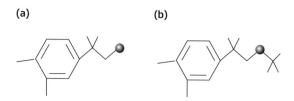

Figure 3.10 (a) The structure of noradrenaline. (b) The structure of salbutamol.

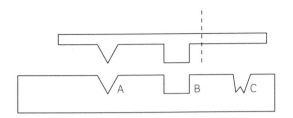

Figure 3.11 How does a receptor blocker work?

the β-receptors in the heart so that noradrenaline and adrenaline cannot occupy them. Since these chemicals make the heart beat stronger and faster, the effect of beta-blockers is to make the heart beat more gently and rather slower, thereby lowering the blood pressure.

Another possibility is that the drug may bind and produce an effect, but not as powerful an effect as another drug, even at high concentrations. For example, the drug buprenorphine binds to the same receptors as morphine, but does not produce the same degree of effect. It is described as a **partial agonist**.

For the sake of completeness, we should mention that there are drugs known as inverse agonists. These bind to receptors and produce the opposite effect to agonists. For example, benzodiazepines are agonists at some brain receptors where they reduce anxiety, but there are experimental drugs that appear to act at the same receptors and cause anxiety. These are inverse agonists. A fuller description of inverse agonists is beyond the scope of this book but a useful summary including some examples is given by Khilnani and Khilnani (2011).

Review of drug-receptor interactions

- Receptors are areas on the surface of organs where natural chemicals will attach to produce a response.
- Drugs with a similar structure can mimic the natural chemicals and also elicit a response. These are called agonists.
- Some drugs do not fit precisely enough to trigger a response, but are able to attach to the receptor, preventing other chemicals or drugs from doing so. These are called antagonists or blockers.

Selectivity, affinity, and efficacy

These terms are used about the drug-receptor interaction and are sometimes confused.

Selectivity indicates that drugs act in particular places, where the appropriate receptors are located. For example, the natural chemical acetylcholine is found within a lot of nerve junctions, but its antagonist atropine only inhibits some of those actions. It interferes with the actions of acetylcholine on smooth muscles, but not on skeletal muscles. This is because acetylcholine acts on more than one type of receptor, whereas atropine is specific for only one variety. The more selective a drug is, the more its action is restricted to particular sites. Some of the side effects of drugs may be caused because the drug acts at receptors outside its target organs, and hence is not sufficiently selective. For example, the beta-blocker propranolol is intended to act on the heart, but it can precipitate asthma attacks in susceptible individuals, because it is not specific enough; it also blocks β-receptors in the airways and so causes bronchoconstriction.

Efficacy measures how likely the drug is to produce a response once it has engaged with the receptor. Drugs with higher efficacy are more likely to produce the effect that we see. It is therefore a measure of activity.

Affinity is a measure of the strength of the binding between the drug and the receptor. If two drugs are competing for the same receptor, the drug with higher affinity is more likely to displace the other.

It follows from these definitions, that agonists possess affinity and efficacy. They will bind to receptors and produce a response. By contrast, antagonists possess affinity but not efficacy. They can bind to receptors, but nothing happens as a result. Partial agonists have affinity but only limited efficacy because although they can bind (affinity) they do not produce a full response (so they have reduced efficacy). Note that a drug that acts as a partial agonist at one receptor may act as a full agonist at another, so when we describe a drug as a partial agonist, we should explain which receptor we have in mind.

Classifying antagonism

The connection between a drug and its receptor is not permanent. If it were, each receptor could only be used once, and a physiological effect, once produced, would last forever. Instead, we should think of the bond as being made and broken many times a second. A snapshot might show that at any given time a lot of receptors are occupied, but a similar picture a split second later would show occupation of a similar number, but not the same receptors.

You can picture this binding and separating as rather like a game of musical chairs. At the moment that the music stops, some of the chairs—the receptors—will be occupied, while some of the children—the drug molecules—will not have found a chair. But what happens if more than one drug is competing for the same receptors?

Our analogy helps us to see the answer. Suppose some of the children are in blue tops, while the others are in red. Unless there is something different about the children, our best guess for the outcome will be that the proportions occupying the chairs when the music stops will be related to the proportions wearing each colour. If there are two blues for each red, the likeliest result is that two chairs will be occupied by children in blue for each one filled by a child in red. So it is with drugs. When drugs compete for receptors, the likely outcome is determined by their relative concentrations, and if we want to affect the result, we can do so by introducing more of the drug we want to favour.

We can see an example of this in the treatment of opiate overdoses. If a drug misuser overdoses on morphine or a similar drug, we can give naloxone. Naloxone is an antagonist at the main opioid receptor sites and is effective because its affinity for the sites is much higher than that of morphine. In our analogy we said 'unless there is something different', and that is exactly the case here, because naloxone is much less willing to detach from the receptor than morphine, so even with equal concentrations of naloxone and morphine, naloxone gets more than its fair share of receptors. With sufficient naloxone in place, the morphine is displaced from the receptors which it has attached to and cannot cause the respiratory depression that places patients in immediate danger from morphine overdose. This is an example of **competitive antagonism**. Naloxone antagonizes the effect of morphine by competing for the same receptors.

There is an additional complication to treating morphine overdose with naloxone that is worth noting. The half-life of naloxone is around 60–90 minutes, whereas that of morphine is at least an hour longer. As a result, when the naloxone is metabolized and its effect wears off, there will still be morphine in the patient's blood that can now reach the receptors and cause the adverse effects we were trying to prevent. It is therefore important that whenever we try to counter the effect of a drug or poison by giving a competitive antidote, we ensure that we repeat the antidote dosage until the original drug has been metabolized.

The alternative to competitive antagonism is **non-competitive antagonism**. In this case one drug counters the effect of another drug or a natural chemical, but not by competing for the same receptors. For example, if a patient has taken a tablet which causes a rise in blood pressure, they may be given a diuretic (water tablet) to cause them to lose water quickly and thereby lower the blood pressure again. This is not competitive antagonism, because the diuretic acts at a different site to the drug that caused the problem.

Antagonists can also be divided into **reversible**, **irreversible**, and **pseudoirreversible**. When we described the drug-receptor bond we spoke of the bond being made and broken repeatedly. This is reversible antagonism, because the drug separates (the word 'dissociates' is normally used) from the receptor readily. Some drugs do not dissociate so easily, and a few will form stable chemical bonds that cannot be broken. This produces irreversible antagonism, because even if an antidote is available once the bonds have been made it is difficult to remove the drug. Pseudoirreversible antagonism occurs when the dissociation is so slow that to all intents and purposes it can be treated as not happening. The antiviral drug maraviroc acts as a pseudoirreversible antagonist at a receptor. (Pullen et al, 2006).

Potency and efficacy

These are related concepts but must not be confused.

If drug A has the same effect as drug B at lower concentrations, drug A is more potent than drug B. For example, when we compare the anti-inflammatory drugs ibuprofen and diclofenac, we may see that patients need 400 mg ibuprofen to produce a similar effect to 50 mg diclofenac, which means diclofenac is more potent.

However, the manufacturers can compensate for differences in potency by putting more or less drug in each tablet or capsule, so this is relatively unimportant for patients. What is much more important is the maximum effect that the drug can achieve in a patient, when all the relevant receptors are filled.

If two drugs occupy the same number of receptors on a tissue, and one drug elicits a greater biological response than the other drug then that drug has greater efficacy. **Intrinsic activity** is sometimes used to express this.

Review of potency, efficacy, and affinity

- Potency measures the effectiveness of a given amount of drug. Measuring the potency allows us to compare the power of different drugs when the same quantity is given. However, in clinical practice the amount of similar drugs in a dose is not the same, making potency comparisons pointless.
- Efficacy measures how effectively the drug can produce a response when it fully occupies its target receptors.
- Affinity describes the likelihood that a drug will combine with a given receptor.

Alternative mechanisms

Interaction with receptors is not the only way in which medicines can affect the body. Others include:

- Blocking the action of specific enzymes
- Inhibiting cell transport mechanisms
- Acting on invading organisms.

Enzyme blockers

We have already noted that some medicines induce or inhibit enzymes. Inhibition of enzymes is the mode of action of some classes of drug. One of the best-known

of these groups is the angiotensin converting enzyme inhibitors, or ACE inhibitors. To understand these we must first understand what the enzyme does.

The liver secretes a protein, angiotensinogen. This is acted upon by renin released by the kidney. Renin breaks the angiotensinogen molecule to produce angiotensin I, an inactive compound. When the body detects that the blood pressure needs to be increased, it releases angiotensin-converting enzyme, which converts the inactive angiotensin I to a highly active form, angiotensin II. This increases blood pressure by increasing the amount of salt and water that the body retains, as well as causing blood vessels to constrict.

In a patient with hypertension (high blood pressure) we need to prevent the action of angiotensin-converting enzyme. The ACE inhibitors do this, blocking the production of angiotensin II. You will find a list of ACE inhibitors in section 2.5.5.1 of your *BNF*.

A number of our frequently used medicines are enzyme inhibitors. Table 3.2 lists a few of them.

Transport or uptake inhibitors

There are a number of classes of drug that interfere with the movement of chemicals within the body. Here we will give a couple of examples.

The selective serotonin re-uptake inhibitors (SSRIs) are used as anti-depressants. They act at the junction between two nerve fibres, where there is a gap or synapse. The signal which has passed down one nerve fibre is transmitted to the other by messenger chemicals such as serotonin that are released into the gap, migrate to the end of the receiving nerve, and produce a new signal. The messenger molecule is then reabsorbed by the nerve that released it. In depression, it is thought that the amounts of serotonin released are not adequate to produce a satisfactory signal. The SSRIs prevent that reuptake, leaving it in the synaptic cleft for longer and allowing it to build up if stimulation continues. You will find the SSRIs in section 4.3.3 of your *BNF*.

An alternative mechanism is to interfere with the transport of chemicals. The circulatory system is very dependent on the movement of calcium ions. These

Table 3.2 Some common enzyme inhibitors.

Enzyme inhibited	Drug class or typical drug	BNF section	Use/indication
Angiotensin converting enzyme	ACE inhibitors	2.5.5.1	Hypertension
Cyclo-oxygenase II	NSAIDs	10.1.1	Analgesia
Dihydrofolate reductase	Methotrexate	8.1.3	Acute lymphoblastic leukaemia
HMG CoA reductase	Statins	2.12	Lowering LDL cholesterol
Phosphodiesterase	Sildenafil	7.4.5	Erectile dysfunction
Topoisomerase II	Cytotoxic antibiotics	8.1.2	Leukaemia and lymphoma
Transpeptidase	Penicillins	5.1.1	Antibacterial
Vitamin K epoxide reductase	Warfarin	2.8.2	Anticoagulant

ACE, angiotensin converting enzyme; LDL, low-density lipoprotein; NSAID, non-steroidal anti-inflammatory drug.

pass through special openings in cardiac muscle and blood vessels called voltage-gated calcium channels (VGCCs). When an electrical impulse passes through the tissues, these channels open to allow calcium to flow through. Calcium increases the contractility of the heart and narrows the arteries, both of which raise the blood pressure. A group of drugs called calcium channel blockers prevent these channels opening. In turn, calcium does not enter and hence the force of the heart beat is reduced and the arteries relax, causing blood pressure to fall. Some of the drugs in this family have more effect on the heart, and are therefore preferred in the treatment of angina, whereas others are used in hypertension. Some, like nifedipine, will do both, though the dosage required may differ. The calcium channel blockers are described in section 2.6.2 of the *BNF*.

Interference with invading organisms

It was noted in Table 3.2 that penicillin interferes with an enzyme. That enzyme is needed by certain bacteria to construct their cell walls. When penicillin binds to it to render it useless, the bacteria cannot construct new walls and therefore cannot reproduce.

Another example of interference with reproductive processes is the antiviral drug aciclovir, which is used to combat infections by herpes viruses. Aciclovir is actually a prodrug. It resembles the molecule guanosine, which is one of the building blocks used to manufacture deoxyribonucleic acid (DNA). Aciclovir is acted upon by viral enzymes to convert it into acyclo-guanosine monophosphate (acyclo-GMP), which is then converted by the host's enzymes into a triphosphate (acyclo-GTP). This triphosphate is used by DNA polymerase enzymes in the virus to construct new DNA for daughter virus cells, but because aciclovir differs from guanosine the DNA that is manufactured is useless for making new virus particles.

Adverse drug reactions

A weed may just be a plant that is growing in the wrong place. In the same way, an adverse drug reaction (sometimes called a side-effect) may simply be an effect that we did not want for that particular patient. For example, many traditional antihistamines cause drowsiness, which we regard as an adverse reaction, but those that cause most drowsiness are sold as over the counter sleep aids. It is therefore hard to describe drowsiness as a side-effect of those antihistamines, when that is exactly the result we were taking them for. For this reason, the term 'side-effect' is less used than it used to be, and we prefer 'adverse drug reaction', which simply describes what is seen, as it affects the patient.

Adverse drug reactions (or ADRs) may arise because the drug affects a receptor outside its main target organ. For example, the anti-asthma drug salbutamol is used in an inhaler to try to limit its effects to the airways, but in large doses enough may be absorbed to allow it to cause tremors in skeletal muscles. Given by infusion it can also be used to reduce uterine contractions in premature labour. Since an infusion reaches most parts of the body, ADRs are more likely with the infusion than with the inhaler.

These unintended effects are not always agonist effects. Sometimes a drug is an agonist at one receptor, but a blocker at another. An example is buprenorphine, which is used as a painkiller and in the management of substance misuse. It is a partial agonist at two types of opioid receptor but an antagonist at another one.

It can be helpful to divide adverse drug reactions into two major groups—Type A (augmented) and Type B (bizarre)—Table 3.3 describes the main differences between the two.

Type A adverse reactions are much more common. The effect seen is related to the known action of the drug, and is usually in proportion to the dose that has been given. They are called augmented because the reaction is normal in type, but bigger in size than we expect. Sometimes the reaction arises because the patient is unusually sensitive to normal doses, perhaps because they have enzymes that do not effectively metabolize it in the usual way. These reactions are rarely fatal, because their cause is easily determined and the right treatment is normally clear—we discontinue the drug causing the problem or give supportive measures until the effect wears off. When this cannot be done,

we may give another treatment to ease the adverse reaction. For instance, many patients feel nauseous when given anti-cancer drugs, so in anticipation of that feeling they may be offered treatment for nausea when their anti-cancer treatment is given.

Type B adverse reactions are much less common, but are more likely to be reported in newspapers because they are dramatic and unexpected. They are unrelated to known pharmacology, which is why they are unexpected and why they are called bizarre. They may not be dose-related, because even tiny doses produce severe effects, and they are idiosyncratic—that is, they are flukes related to the individual patient, and may not occur in other patients. Since they are not predictable, and it may not be immediately clear that the effect we are seeing is related to a particular drug, they may be life threatening because the best treatment may not be obvious at the time. Anaphylactic shock following a treatment would usually be classed as a Type B reaction.

Once sufficient evidence accumulates, we may discover the cause of a type B reaction, in which event it becomes type A because we now know what the cause is and hence predict when it may occur. Moreover, knowing the cause, we are more likely to be able to treat cases which occur. In the section on pharmacogenetics there was mention of a small group of patients who cannot metabolize suxamethonium. Their adverse reactions were originally type B reactions, because they were life threatening and limited to a small subgroup of patients. Since the underlying pharmacology was not known, treating the reaction was very difficult. Once the cause was discovered it became easier to

Table 3.3 Adverse drug reactions.

Type A, Augmented	Type B, Bizarre
more common type	unexpected or unpredictable
relates to known pharmacology	unrelated to known pharmacology
usually dose-related	not usually dose-related
may involve exaggerated effect of standard doses	idiosyncratic
rarely fatal	rare but may be life-threatening

support these patients until they had metabolized sufficient drug for the effects to wear off.

Another example is that of long-action antipsychotic injections. One such injection had the drug dissolved in oil and injected into the patient's buttock. This made the injection into a slow release form and meant that the patients did not need such frequent injections. One such patient had a serious reaction to the injection and required intensive care. This was a type B reaction, because it was unclear why this should happen to him and not to all the others, but in time it was discovered that the injection contained traces of peanut oil, and the patient had reacted in this way because he was allergic to peanuts.

The onset of an adverse drug reaction may be immediate—as in anaphylaxis—or delayed by months or years. Long-term or high-dose use of antipsychotic drugs may produce tardive dyskinesia—jerky, uncoordinated body movements - years after treatment started. ADRs may be reversible or irreversible. Even if they are reversible, recovery may not be immediate on discontinuation of the drug, and sometimes does not happen at all.

Review of adverse drug reactions

- Adverse drug reactions are unwanted effects of a drug given at normal doses. They may be clinically unimportant, but some are life threatening.

- They arise when a drug has an exaggerated effect in a patient, or when the drug acts on a body system which was not its primary target.

- They may be type A, in which the drug produces its normal effect but to an exaggerated degree, or type B when the drug produces an unexpected result.

- Some adverse reactions resolve when the drug is withdrawn, but in a minority of cases they may persist after withdrawal.

- All suspected adverse reactions should be reported to senior colleagues and ultimately through the yellow card system (see section on the national reporting and learning service and the yellow card system, Chapter 2) in accordance with local procedures.

Drug interactions

A drug interaction is the modification of the effect of a drug brought about by another drug concurrently administered. There are also food-drug interactions and interactions between drugs and chemicals, both environmental and internal—the body's own chemicals such as hormones. They may be trivial or serious, can be exacerbated by a patient's other diseases, and the modifying agent may not be something that the patient thinks of as a drug. Some parts of our diet can interfere with drug action, while patients may buy health supplements that can affect the actions of their prescribed medication, but may forget to include these when listing the medicines they take.

There are a number of ways in which drug interactions can come about. These include:

- Interference with metabolism
- Alteration of absorption
- Displacement of bound drug
- Additive or synergistic effect
- Antagonistic effect
- Alteration of excretion rate
- Disturbance in electrolyte levels.

These can be divided into pharmacokinetic and pharmacodynamic interactions.

Quiz

Based on the earlier part of this chapter, you should be able to divide the bullet point list of drug interactions into those which are caused by changes in pharmacokinetics, and those which are caused by pharmacodynamic changes.

Answers can be found at the end of the chapter.

Pharmacodynamic drug interactions

Pharmacodynamic drug interactions occur between drugs with similar or antagonistic pharmacological effects. If they are similar, they produce an enhanced effect, whereas antagonistic actions may to some extent cancel each other out. Not all drug interactions are unwanted, and we may use interactions to produce a better effect with two drugs than either drug could produce on its own. For example, when treating high blood pressure, it is common to give a low dose of a diuretic medicine and a small dose of a calcium-channel blocker. These work well together to reduce blood pressure in different ways. If either were used in large doses the effect might be the same but the side effects would probably be difficult for patients to tolerate.

Pharmacodynamic interactions may therefore involve either competition at receptor sites, or separate actions on the same physiological system. They are usually predictable if the pharmacology of the drugs involved is known, and because they are related to that pharmacology, they will occur to some extent in most patients who receive that particular combination of drugs. Moreover, since the effects produced by a drug are shared by others in its family, the interaction is normally a **class effect**—that is, it occurs with all the drugs in that family rather than being specific to a single member.

Pharmacokinetic drug interactions

We can contrast these with pharmacokinetic drug interactions. These occur when one drug alters the absorption, distribution, metabolism, or excretion of another, thus increasing or reducing the amount of drug available to produce its pharmacological effects. While some of these are quite predictable, others may not be. For example, colestyramine is a medicine used to reduce hypercholesterolaemia (high cholesterol levels in the blood). It does this by binding to bile acids in the intestine. However, its ability to bind is not selective, and it may bind to other medicines present in the intestines. This feature is used in some cases of drug overdose, when colestyramine may be given to try to absorb medicine before it enters the blood. Similarly, the fact that two drugs are metabolized by the same enzyme, which means that one will have to wait until the enzyme system becomes free, thus leaving it longer in the body unchanged and active, may or may not be known.

A good example is the interaction of some drugs with grapefruit juice. One such drug is felodipine, which is used to treat high blood pressure. Grapefruit juice contains substances called furanocoumarins, which inhibit the action of the enzyme CYP3A4. This inhibition means that drugs like felodipine that are metabolized by CYP3A4 will be able to reach the circulation in greater quantities, leading to higher blood levels, which can potentially cause adverse effects. This is not a small effect; in one trial when patients were given 250 ml of grapefruit juice the peak blood level of felodipine increased by 89% (Goosen et al, 2004).

Since the pharmacokinetics of a drug depend to a large degree on the individual patient, these interactions may not be universal. Some patients will experience no interaction, while others may suffer considerably.

Unlike pharmacodynamic drug interactions, pharmacokinetic interactions do not necessarily show class effects. Differences in metabolic pathways, enzymes involved, half-life, and chemical properties mean that drugs in the same group do not share pharmacokinetic interactions, though obviously the closer the relationship between drugs, the more likely it is that they will. For example, the proton pump inhibitors lansoprazole and omeprazole are quite similar in structure and are used for the same purposes, but differ in their interactions to some extent. Lansoprazole has less effect on the metabolism of tacrolimus than omeprazole has. (Hosohata et al, 2009)

Review of drug interactions

- Drug interactions may be pharmacokinetic or pharmacodynamic. In pharmacokinetic interactions, one drug or substance interferes with the way in which another is absorbed, distributed, metabolized, or excreted.

- In pharmacodynamic interactions, one drug or substance acts on the body system to oppose or enhance the effect of another.

- Not all interactions are unwelcome. When two drugs produce the same effect via different mechanisms it becomes possible to achieve a better result than could be achieved by using either drug alone.

Complementary medicines

There is a lot of interest in complementary medicines, and a lot of misunderstanding about them. Patients sometimes think that complementary medicines are more 'natural' and that natural medicines have a reduced level of risk. Of course, strychnine, salmonella, and botulinum are all natural products, but definitely not without risk!

There can be no doubt that herbal medicines may be effective, because a number of drugs used in conventional medicine have a herbal basis and their efficacy has been proven. Digoxin was originally used in the form of foxglove, the plant that contains it; opiates were developed from poppy extracts; aloes and senna-pods were used as laxatives. There is good evidence that guaraná improves concentration (Kennedy et al, 2004) and that saw palmetto, which contains compounds very similar to some of our synthetic drugs, is effective in the milder forms of prostate disease (Gordon and Shaughnessy, 2003). The difficulty with using raw plants is that the amount of active ingredient in individual plants may vary considerably, so for consistency of effect the plant must be processed to standardize the content.

Perhaps the current herbal product with most evidence for its efficacy is St John's wort, which is used as an antidepressant (Linde et al, 2009). Preparations on sale differ markedly in declared content, and consumers must be careful to check whether the dose is given in terms of extract or whole plant, since the content described on the label may be misleading without this information.

In general, if a product has a medicinal action, it can interact with another drug and can cause adverse reactions. Some herbal or complementary medicines have a significant number of important drug interactions.

Again St John's wort is a leading example. It causes induction of some liver enzymes, leading to reduced blood concentrations of a large range of drugs. It reduces the contraceptive effect of oestrogens, for example, and should therefore not be used by women who are taking oestrogen-containing oral contraceptives, See Appendix 1 of the *BNF* for a complete list of interactions with St John's wort.

For this reason when patients are asked to give a list of their drugs they must be asked specifically if they are taking any herbal or alternative medicines. Students with an interest in this area may find Barnes et al (2007) helpful.

Summary

An understanding of elementary pharmacology helps nurses to support patients in gaining the most benefit from their medication. This chapter has described basic pharmacokinetics, pharmacodynamics, and pharmacogenetics. It has given an introduction to the pharmacokinetic phases of absorption, distribution, metabolism, and excretion and described how the body handles medicines, noting that our genetic makeup can cause variation in the way medicines are handled. It has also outlined some of the ways in which medicines act and introduced the key concepts of receptors, agonists, and antagonists. Together these allow us to predict adverse drug reactions and interactions and mitigate them, enhancing the benefits of the medicines and the safety of our patients.

Further reading

Students who wish to develop their knowledge of pharmacokinetics further may find *Clinical Pharmacokinetics* by Dhillon and Kostrzewski (2006) useful. Appendix 1 of the *BNF* contains many drug interactions, though it does not generally explain how they come about. The most comprehensive source of information is *Stockley's Drug Interactions* (Baxter, 2010). Each interaction is described with its mechanism where these are known, and the likely clinical importance is also discussed. There is a pocket companion which costs much less but obviously gives less information. A recent innovation has been *Stockley's Herbal Medicines Interactions* (Williamson et al, 2009) which describes the evidence base for interactions involving herbal medicines. These are not books that the pre-registration nurse would be expected to own, but it would be useful to look for them in your library and understand the type of information that can be found in them.

References

Armstrong CJ, and Wilson TS (1995), Systemic absorption of vancomycin, *Journal of Clinical Pathology*, 48; 689. Available at http://www.ncbi.nlm.nih.gov/pmc/articles/PMC502731/?page=1 (accessed 8 July 2012).

Ashraful Alam M, Uddin R, and Haque S (2008), Protein binding interaction of warfarin and acetaminophen in presence of arsenic and of the biological system, *Bangladesh J Pharmacol* 3: 49–54

Barnes J, Anderson L A, and Phillipson JD (2007), *Herbal Medicines* (3rd ed). Pharmaceutical Press, London.

Baxter K (2010) *Stockley's Drug Interactions*. Pharmaceutical Press, London.

BNF see Joint Formulary Committee.

Cruickshank JM, Neil-Dwyer G, Cameron MM, and McAinsh J (1980), Beta-Adrenoreceptor-blocking agents and the blood-brain barrier. *Clinical Science (London)*. 1980, 59 (S6):453S–455S.

Dever LL (2000), *Emerging Antibiotic Resistance in Nosocomial Pathogens*, available at: http://www.rtmagazine.com/issues/articles/2000-08_07.asp (accessed 5 June 2012).

Dharmarajan TS, Adiga GU, and Norkus EP (2003) Vitamin B_{12} deficiency: Recognizing subtle symptoms in older adults. *Geriatrics* 58: 30–38. Available at: http://geriatrics.modernmedicine.com/geriatrics/data/articlestandard//geriatrics/122003/50225/article.pdf (accessed 8 July 2012).

Dhillon S, and Kostrzewski A, (eds) (2006) *Clinical Pharmacokinetics*. Pharmaceutical Press: London.

Gasche Y, Daali Y, Fathi M, Chiappe A, Cottini S, Dayer P, and Desmeules J (2004) Codeine Intoxication Associated with Ultrarapid CYP2D6 Metabolism, *New England Journal of Medicine* 351: 2827–2831.

Goldstein JA, Ishizaki T, Chiba K, de Morais SMF, Bell D, Krahn PM, et al (1997), Frequencies of the defective CYP2C19 alleles responsible for the mephenytoin poor metabolizer phenotype in various Oriental, Caucasian, Saudi Arabian and American Black populations. *Pharmacogenetics* 7 :59–64.

Goosen TC, Cillié D, Bailey DG, Yu C, He K, Hollenberg PF, et al (2004). Bergamottin contribution to the grapefruit juice-felodipine interaction and disposition in humans, *Clinical Pharmacology and Therapeutics*, 76: 607–617

Gordon AE and Shaughnessy AF (2003), Saw palmetto for prostate disorders, *American Family Physician*, 67: 1281–1283.

Hosohata K, Masuda S, Katsura T, Takada Y, Kaido T, Ogura Y, et al (2009), Impact of Intestinal *CYP2C19* Genotypes on the Interaction between Tacrolimus and Omeprazole, but not Lansoprazole. In Adult Living-Donor Liver Transplant Patients, *Drug Metabolism and Disposition*, 37: 821–826.

Ingelman-Sundberg M, (2005), Genetic polymorphisms of cytochrome *P450* 2D6 (CYP2D6): clinical consequences, evolutionary aspects and functional diversity, *The Pharmacogenomics Journal*, 5; 6–13.

Jambhekar S and Breen PJ (2009), *Basic pharmacokinetics*. Pharmaceutical Press: London.

Joint Formulary Committee (2012), *British National Formulary* (64th ed). London: BMJ Group and Pharmaceutical Press.

Kennedy DO, Haskell CF, Wesnes KA, et al. (2004), Improved cognitive performance in human volunteers following administration of guarana (*Paullinia cupana*) extract: comparison and interaction with Panax ginseng. *Pharmacology Biochemistry and Behavior*, 79: 401–411.

Khilnani G and Khilnani AK (2011), Inverse agonism and its therapeutic significance. Indian *Journal of Pharmacology* 43: 492–501. Available at: http://www.ijp-online.com/text.asp?2011/43/5/492/84947 (accessed 8 July 2012).

Larsen RH, Nielsen F, Sørensen JA, and Nielsen JB (2003), Dermal Penetration of Fentanyl: Inter- and Intra-individual Variations. *Pharmacology and Toxicology*, 93: 244–248.

Liao JK (2007), Safety and Efficacy of Statins in Asians, *American Journal Cardiology*, 99: 410–414.

Linde K, Berner MM, and Kriston L (2009), St. John's wort for treating depression, *Cochrane Database of Systematic Reviews* 2008, Issue 4. Art. No.: CD000448. DOI: 10.1002/14651858.CD000448.pub3. Available at: http://onlinelibrary.wiley.com/doi/10.1002/14651858.CD000448.pub3/pdf/standard (accessed 4 May 2012).

Lomas C (2009), Nurse Prescribing: The next steps. Available at: http://www.nursingtimes.net/nursing-practice/clinical-specialisms/prescribing/nurse-prescribing-the-next-steps/5003904.article (accessed 22 May 2012).

MacFadyen RJ, Meredith PA, and Elliott HL (1993), Enalapril clinical pharmacokinetics and pharmacokinetic-pharmacodynamic relationships. An overview. *Clinical Pharmacokinetics*. 25: 274–282.

Medicines and Healthcare products Regulatory Agency (2008), *Fentanyl Patches: Serious and Fatal Overdose from*

Dosing Errors, Accidental Exposure, and Inappropriate Use, Drug Safety Update 2(2). London: MHRA.

Pullen S, Sale H, Napier C, Mansfield R, and Holbrook M, *Maraviroc (UK–427,857) is a Slowly Reversible Antagonist at the Human CCR5 in a CRE-Luciferase Reporter Gene Assay*, at: http://www.retroconference.org/2006/PDFs/504.pdf (accessed 1 may 2012).

Sweetman S (ed.) (2011), *Martindale: The Complete Drug Reference* (37th ed), London: Pharmaceutical Press.

Williamson E, Driver S, and Baxter K (2009), *Stockley's Herbal Medicines Interactions*. London: Pharmaceutical Press.

Wu JY, Kim JJ, Reddy R, Wang WM, Graham DY, Kwon DH (2005), Tetracycline-Resistant Clinical Helicobacter pylori Isolates with and without Mutations in 16S rRNA-Encoding Genes, *Antimicrobial Agents and Chemotherapy*, 49: 578–583.

Quiz answers

Interference with metabolism—pharmacokinetic interaction.

Alteration of absorption—pharmacokinetic interaction.

Displacement of bound drug—pharmacokinetic interaction.

Additive or synergistic effect—pharmacodynamic interaction.

Antagonistic effect—pharmacodynamic interaction.

Alteration of excretion rate—pharmacokinetic interaction.

Disturbance in electrolyte levels—pharmacodynamic interaction.

4 Pharmaceutics and Routes of Drug Administration

CHAPTER CONTENTS

- Routes of administration: pros and cons
- Oral administration
- Enteral administration
- Rectal and vaginal routes

- Respiratory route
- Injections and infusions
- Topical or transdermal
- Summary

LEARNING OUTCOMES

By the end of this chapter you should understand:

- The range of routes via which medicines can be given
- The formulations of medicines that are commonly used
- How the route selected can affect a drug's properties.

Routes of administration: pros and cons

All medicines must be administered as prescribed and following the manufacturers' guidance. The main aim of medicines management is to achieve the desired therapeutic effect for the patient. In order to do this you need to:

- give the correct medicine,
- at the correct dose,
- to the correct person,
- in the correct formulation,
- by the correct route, and
- at the appropriate time intervals.

This has already been mentioned in Chapter 1.

You must consider the dosage, the patient's weight where appropriate, **method of administration**, route, and timing (NMC, 2008a). Equally, when preparing to administer any medication, it is important to follow the principles of standard precautions (Glasper et al, 2009). For example, when administering oral medicines you should first wash your hands and then use a non-touch technique to prevent cross infection and to ensure that the drug does not cause you any harm.

The way in which a drug is administered will affect the rate and extent of absorption. There are three basic routes for administration of medicines: enteral (via the GI tract), parenteral, and topical (Lilley et al,

Exercise 4.1

List all of the ways of giving medicines that you know.
   Highlight those that you have used for the administration of medicines.
   Consider what you needed to know about the medicine and the route prior to administration.

2007). However, within these a variety of methods can be used.

Medicines are introduced into the body via many routes, which include:

- Oral
- Enteral (via a nasogastric or gastrostomy tube)
- Rectal
- Vaginal
- Respiratory
- Intradermal injection
- Subcutaneous injection
- Intramuscular injection
- Intravenous injection
- Infusions
- Intrathecal and epidural
- Topical/transdermal.

Exercise 4.2

Consider the list.
   What do these terms mean to you?
   What do these terms mean to patients?
   Think of one advantage, and one disadvantage, for each route.
   Think of a patient to whom you have administered medicines by one or more of these routes.

The aim of treatment is to deliver the optimal amount of medication to the part of the body where it will act. Usually we would like the concentration of drug to reach therapeutic levels (the level at which it exerts its medicinal action) as quickly as possible. This usually means that we want a particular level of drug in the bloodstream. The quickest route to achieve therapeutic levels of drugs is the intravenous route, because

the drugs are delivered directly into the bloodstream and levels rise as soon as the drug is given. However, this may not be the most appropriate route for the administration of medicines for many reasons. Each route has its own advantages and disadvantages and certain drugs must be administered by one route only, while others may be given by more than one route.

Oral administration

The oral route (i.e. given by mouth) is the most common route used for administering medicines and is usually the safest, least expensive, and most convenient, especially if the medicine is available over the counter (Scott and McGrath, 2008). However, some drugs cannot be administered orally if, for example, they would be destroyed by digestion. Also, the oral route may not be appropriate if, for example, the patient is feeling nauseated or is unable to co-operate.

Oral medicines come in many forms, including tablets, capsules, and suspensions, and generally can only be given if the patient is conscious and able to swallow. Some oral medication has an unpleasant taste but may be tolerated if followed by a flavoured drink.

Tablet, capsule, or pill?

These words are sometimes used interchangeably, but they have different definitions. Very few true pills are made today. The active ingredient is mixed with a carrier paste rather like dough and rolled out into a sausage shape, which is then cut. Each pill is rolled to give it a smooth, oval shape like a rugby ball, and may then be coated. However, pills are generally quite fragile and there is a limit to the amount of drug that one pill can hold without becoming too big to swallow comfortably.

A tablet is made in a similar way but compacted under pressure in a mould. This pressure means that a tablet is smaller than a pill containing a similar amount of drug. It is also harder and therefore less likely to crumble. The stamping motion that produces the tablet gives it a characteristic shape, flatter than a pill; though the actual shape and cross-sectional appearance are determined by the way the mould and stamp are shaped.

Soluble or dispersible tablets are made in the same way but contain substances that will effervesce when placed in water. This disrupts the tablet and causes it to break apart. Strictly, soluble tablets are those that dissolve completely to give a clear solution. Dispersible tablets give a cloudy liquid. You may have noticed that many brands of aspirin do not give a clear liquid, but have a grey or milky appearance when dissolved. Under a microscope you can see tiny fragments of insoluble material. When these tablets are taken you must be careful to swirl the contents and may have to rinse the container and allow the patient to swallow the contents, because powdered tablet may stick to the cup.

Tablets take some time to dissolve in the stomach, so the medications within them will generally take 30–60 minutes to begin to act. By coating the tablets with a special **gastroresistant** lacquer, it is possible to avoid dissolution in the stomach where gastric acid may damage the active ingredients and thus deliver the medicine to the small intestine, reducing the risk of damage to the gastric mucosa and, in some cases, delivering the medication directly to its site of action. For prolonged action, the medication may be incorporated in a modified-release tablet. Some of these have extra coating to slow dissolution, while others have tiny pores through which the medication slowly escapes. A third type consists of coated granules embedded in a medium that will dissolve quickly. In this way it may be possible to give a medicine only once a day, which the patient may prefer. These coated or matrix tablets must not be crushed, or their special properties will be lost.

Capsules consist of a casing usually made in two parts, often from gelatin, though alternatives may be available that can be taken by vegetarians. The medicine is in powder or granule form inside the capsule. These may give a slightly quicker onset of action, because once the casing is dissolved in the stomach, the powder is soon absorbed, but again, the lack of compacting means that there is a limit to the volume a capsule can contain. As with tablets, the granules within a capsule may themselves be coated to slow their dissolution. When a patient cannot swallow, it may be possible to give them the contents of a capsule mixed with a small amount of liquid. (Figure 4.1 shows a pack of capsules and a pack of pills.)

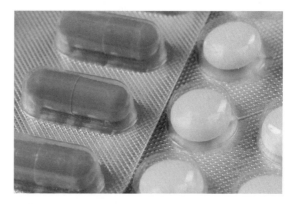

Figure 4.1 Capsules and tablets.
©istockphoto/troninphoto.

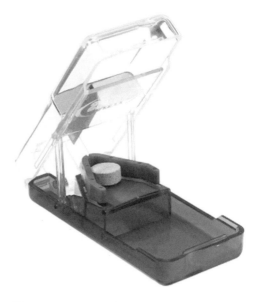

Figure 4.2 A tablet cutter.
Courtesy of Primo Health Ltd.

Some capsules have contents which are either liquids or gels, inside a soft gelatin coating. The soft shell dissolves quickly but may be sensitive to heat. In hot or humid weather these capsules may stick to each other in their container and become unusable.

Nursing considerations when administering oral medicines

You should not break tablets unless they are scored and you use an appropriate tablet cutter to ensure the correct dose (Figure 4.2) (Glasper et al, 2009).

For patients with difficulties taking tablets, soluble or liquid preparations may be available. Some tablets can be reduced to powder in a tablet crusher, which works like a peppermill, but this should only be done in the patient's best interest and with the agreement of a pharmacist in case the crushing changes the properties of the medicine (NMC, 2008a). You should also be aware that in most cases crushing a tablet will mean that it is being used outside the terms of its product licence; it becomes, in effect, an unlicensed medicine.

To achieve maximum absorption most oral medicines should be taken before food since a tablet taken with or just after food will be delayed in entering the small intestine, where most absorption takes place (McGavock, 2004). Certain medicines interact with food, necessitating administration between meals or on an empty stomach. An example of this is oxytetracycline, the absorption of which is reduced if the patient consumes dairy products. Others require the patient to take with food (BNF, 2012), for example non-steroidal anti-inflammatory drugs, due to their potentially damaging effects on the gastrointestinal tract. Check the information leaflets for details of medicines that should be taken with or without food so that you can emphasize the importance to patients. Clearly, the necessity to adhere to these requirements can be a disadvantage for some patients, particularly when some of their medicines must be taken before food, and others are taken with or after it.

Some oral medication will be prescribed in sublingual form, requiring the patient to hold it under the tongue. Similarly, the buccal route means the medication should be placed between the gum and the inside of the mouth. Medication is absorbed more rapidly from oral mucosa and, given in this way, avoids gastric breakdown and absorption, as well as avoiding first pass metabolism in the liver. As we shall see later, glyceryl trinitrate is inactive if swallowed, but is a useful medicine in angina when placed or sprayed under the tongue.

Some laxatives are produced as granules which must be mixed with water before use. These should not be allowed to stand, because the mixture becomes thicker with the passage of time.

In the United Kingdom, liquid medicines are formulated so that a standard dose is usually 5 ml or a multiple of that, and standard medicine spoons are available to measure the dose. No other spoon should be used. A household teaspoon, for example, may contain anything from 4 ml to 8 ml. If a patient needs a large number of spoonfuls at a time, either use an approved medicines' measure (which looks like a little tumbler) or measure the medicine on a 5 ml spoon and pour the measured spoonfuls into a small cup to give to the patient.

If the dose is less than 5 ml, which is often the case for small children, an oral syringe should be used to give the medicine. This looks like an injection syringe, but has no needle and is usually coloured so that it will not be confused with an injection syringe. There may be an adaptor that will fit the neck of the bottle. The syringe is inserted into the adaptor and the bottle can then be turned upside down without risk of spillage so that you can withdraw the right amount of medicine by pulling on the plunger. The syringe is withdrawn from the adaptor (after turning the bottle the right way up!) and the contents can then be gently squirted inside the patient's cheek. Never point the syringe directly at the back of the throat because there is a risk that a patient could choke or inhale the medication.

It is important that patients are given clear information about the way in which oral medication should be administered to ensure effectiveness.

Enteral administration

Enteral administration means the administration of the drug directly into the gastro- intestinal tract. Some patients will have enteral tubes in place and it may be possible for some oral drugs to be administered via this route. Remember that you must always follow instructions as written on the prescription. If using an enteral tube for administering medicines, van den Bernt et al (2006) recommend following these rules:

1 Stop the enteral feeding prior to drug administration.

2 Flush the enteral tube.

3   Generally tablets should not be crushed, as this might change the properties or nature of the drug, but some can (check the manufacturer's guidance and if in doubt, contact your pharmacist). Inappropriate crushing can lead to obstruction of the enteral tube or loss of efficacy. See: **http://www.ismp.org/Tools/DoNotCrush.pdf** and NMC (2008a) *Standards for Medicines Management*.

4   Do not mix different tablets as this might cause an adverse drug reaction.

5   Use dispersible tablets when possible providing they disperse within 2 minutes.

6   Flush after administration.

Rectal and vaginal routes

Enemas and suppositories can be used to deliver medication. Enemas are solutions instilled into the rectum to obtain therapeutic effects or for diagnostic purposes. Suppositories are solid or semi-solid pellets, which melt at body temperature or are dissolved in the mucous secretions of the rectum (Dougherty and Lister, 2008). Medication administered in this way can be used for local or systemic effects as they are relatively rapidly absorbed (Lilley et al, 2007). Many drugs, such as opioids, are well absorbed when administered rectally.

Rectal administration of medication may be used to treat constipation and, in this case, preparation is needed to ensure the patient can easily and quickly access the toilet or commode. The patient should be encouraged to retain the enema or suppositories for

Box 4.1 Glycerin suppositories

Glycerin suppositories begin to dissolve by drawing water from the rectal mucosa. This can cause stinging and discomfort, which can be avoided if you dip the tip of the suppository in water just before insertion. Handle them for as short a time as possible, because the heat from your hands will soften them, even through gloves. Some suppositories are wrapped in clear plastic, which needs removing before use.

the recommended duration stipulated by the manufacturer. For long-term treatment given rectally, patients can be taught to self-administer but this may not always be possible.

Pessaries are solid pellets inserted into the vagina and usually designed to have a local therapeutic action. They are best inserted last thing at night as they can become dislodged (Trounce, 2000). Creams can also be administered vaginally. However, self-administration of a vaginal cream is not easy and a vaginal applicator or extended nozzle should be used if one is available. These allow deeper insertion of the cream and, in the case of the applicator; they help to measure the dose. The applicator is a tube with a plunger in it, rather like a syringe. The tube is filled from the container of cream, inserted gently into the vagina, and then the plunger is pushed upwards, which forces the cream out.

When administering rectal or vaginal medication remember to consider that patients may find this embarrassing and may be anxious about this route of administration. You will need to ensure that a patient's privacy, dignity, and comfort are maintained at all times (Pegram et al, 2008). A chaperone is desirable, not only because the patient may want one, but also because being alone with a patient to perform an intimate act may put you at risk of allegations that you behaved improperly. Without a chaperone, there is no one to support your side of the story.

Respiratory route

Medicines which are available as gases, dry powders, or aerosols, can be administered by inhalation; given by this method they are rapidly absorbed. Nebulization and the use of various inhaler devices allow the inhalation of a range of drugs, which aim to have a localized effect.

Nebulization

This involves the passage of air or oxygen through a solution of a drug, achieving delivery of a fine mist via a mouthpiece or mask. It is important to have the correct particle size, which is best obtained by using an air flow rate of 6–8 litres/minute. This can be delivered using either piped air or oxygen, or through a compressor, commonly known as a nebulizer. Some antibiotics and bronchodilators can be delivered in this way. The use of a nebulizer enables the delivery of larger doses of the medication to the bronchi (Trounce, 2000). If you are using oxygen, always check that the cylinder or outlet can give an adequate flow rate. Piped oxygen in hospitals is usually adequate, but some domestic flow heads are designed to give a constant, low flow. If in doubt, check with the oxygen supplier before trying to nebulize medication in this way.

Inhalers

A variety of inhalers, with or without a spacer device, can be used to deliver medication. Some deliver the drug in aerosol form, while others deliver powder. The concentration achieved at the site of action can be high although the total dose is relatively small. This results in quick and effective symptom management with fewer side effects than experienced with equivalent oral doses (Dougherty and Lister, 2008).

Patients should be able to choose the easiest and most appropriate device to meet their individual needs. It is important as a health care professional to remember to check the individual's technique as, particularly for older people and children, inhalers can be difficult to use effectively (Dougherty and Lister, 2008). When patients are prescribed two puffs at each dose, some will fire the second inhalation too quickly. The next metered dose is stored in a small chamber at the foot of the inhaler which needs time to refill after actuation. If the second puff is taken too quickly, the chamber will only be part-filled, and the patient will receive a reduced dose.

Some inhalers are automatic and are triggered by the patient's inward breath. While this overcomes problems of poor technique, some patients do not like the sudden jet produced. There are also some patients who are unable to inhale sufficiently strongly to trigger an automatic device. Box 4.2 gives more information about steroid inhalers.

Box 4.2 Steroid inhalers

Steroid inhalers may lead the patient to develop oral thrush, because steroid deposited in the mouth suppresses the natural defences which stop infection by fungi that are always present. The best way of preventing this is to encourage patients using steroid inhalers to rinse their mouths with water after use, not forgetting to clean dentures thoroughly. Using a spacer device reduces the pressure of the jet from the inhaler and hence reduces the amount of medicine deposited in the upper airways where it may cause thrush and hoarseness. The spacer may also reduce the need for co-ordination because the aerosol is squirted into a reservoir from which the patient inhales.

Similarly, steroid particles may land on the vocal cords, producing hoarseness. This cannot easily be prevented, but you should watch for signs that it is present and report them to a senior colleague if you see them.

Injections and infusions

Student nurses are only permitted to give subcutaneous and intramuscular injections, under direct supervision, as other routes are regarded as specialized functions that require further training. However, some advantages and disadvantages of other routes are discussed here.

A key disadvantage with medicines given by injection is that it is difficult to reverse the effects once administered (Lavery and Ingram, 2008). Also, the cost of equipment and practitioners' time to prepare medication for administration needs to be considered in addition to the cost of the medicines.

Some patients may have a fear of needles or injections, which could be due to past experiences. In these cases alternative routes or measures to make the procedure less distressing should be considered.

Exercise 4.3

What measures can you think of to make injections less distressing for the patient?
Read on for some answers.

You may have thought about giving up-to-date information about the equipment used and the drug you are going to administer. The distressing experience may have been some time ago, for example, at one time needles were sterilized and reused, which meant that it was possible that they would become blunt and more force would be needed to pierce the skin. Modern needles are disposable and blunt needles are rare today.

Distraction techniques can be useful, as can application of local anaesthetic cream (Baillie, 2005). Use of a local anaesthetic cream may reduce pain at the site of injection. If cream is not available, an ice-pack wrapped in a towel may numb the area temporarily, or firm pressure immediately before the injection is given by squeezing with the thumb may reduce the discomfort. Encouraging the patient to relax by choosing a comfortable position will make the procedure less painful. For some patients, the problem lies in the sight of the needle, and they will co-operate if you keep the needle out of their sight or suggest that they close their eyes. When consent has been given to the injection, patients may even prefer not to know that you are about to give the injection. Some experienced nurses have learned to give injections to patients while talking about something else so that the patient does not expect the needle.

Intradermal injections

This route, into the dermis, provides a local rather than systemic effect. Local anaesthetics can be administered via this route, as well as it being used for diagnostic purposes such as tuberculin testing. The needle should be inserted almost parallel to the skin, keeping the upright bevel visible under the skin. When resistance is felt and a raised bleb is seen then the route is being used correctly (Diggle, 2007). The commonly used site is the medial forearm (Dougherty and Lister, 2008) though, of course, local anaesthetics can be administered anywhere on the surface of the body according to need.

Subcutaneous injections

Injections given via this route, into the fat and connective tissue underneath the dermis, are given usually into the upper arm, thigh, or abdomen (see Figure 4.3). An angle of 90° into a raised skin fold is recommended today, particularly for administration of heparin and insulin (Glasper et al, 2009) (see Figure 4.4). However, for very thin patients it may be necessary to use a 45° angle to ensure the drug is administered to the correct area.

The maximum volume given using this route is 2 ml and only highly soluble drugs may be used to prevent irritation (Workman, 1999). Following injection, the drug enters the capillaries by diffusion or filtration,

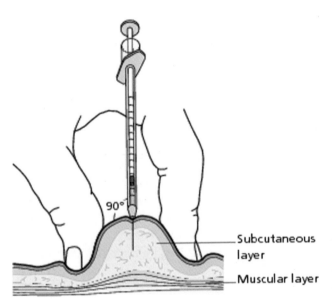

Figure 4.3 A subcutaneous injection at a 90 degree angle.
Reproduced from Endacott, Jevon, and Cooper, *Clinical Nursing Skills, Core and Advanced*, 2009, with permission from Oxford University Press.

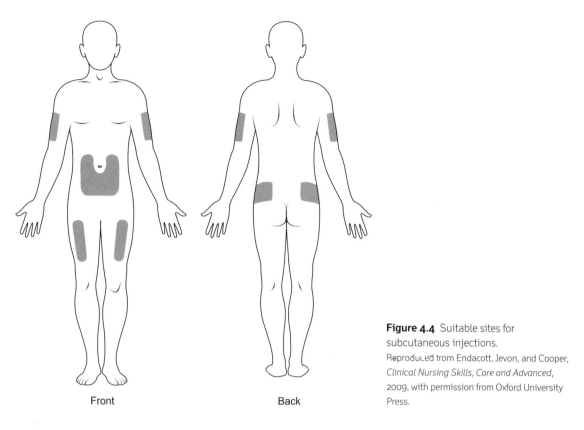

Front   Back

Figure 4.4 Suitable sites for subcutaneous injections.
Reproduced from Endacott, Jevon, and Cooper, *Clinical Nursing Skills, Core and Advanced*, 2009, with permission from Oxford University Press.

providing slow absorption. Patients using this route can be taught to self-administer their medication.

It is good practice not to use the same injection site repeatedly. This may produce problems, particularly with insulin, where the underlying skin structures may be damaged by repeated injection.

Intramuscular injections

Using this route delivers the medication directly into the densest part of the selected muscle, where there are fewer pain-sensing nerves than in the subcutaneous tissue (Hunter, 2007). A number of sites can be used, including mid-deltoid, dorsogluteal, and ventrogluteal. The Z-track technique should always be used to minimize reflux following withdrawal of the needle (Glapser et al, 2009).

Onset of action is typically more rapid than when using the subcutaneous route. However, while drugs may be absorbed quickly following intramuscular injection, the absorption rate depends on blood flow at the injection site. That in turn can be affected by recent exercise, or even heat from a radiator or electric blanket. In older people decreased muscle mass may result in faster absorption of drugs delivered using this route (Perry and Potter, 2004).

Drugs that are not readily soluble can provide sustained action following an intramuscular injection when delivered in suspension form. For example, antipsychotic depot medication is slowly released into the body over a number of weeks to provide maintenance therapy (BNF, 2012).

Intravenous administration

Bioavailability is the proportion of the administered drug that reaches the blood stream and is therefore available for the body to use. Using this route provides 100% **bioavailability** of the drug because, by definition, it all reaches the circulation. It also avoids **first-pass metabolism** i.e. being transported directly to the liver following administration and being partially inactivated there. Medicines delivered in this way have a rapid onset of action. However, intravenous drugs are often more costly than the same medication used orally, and they need to be administered by a trained health care professional. Any nurse administering intravenous drugs must be a registered practitioner who is competent and acting in accordance with the NMC code (2008b).

Administration of intravenous drugs can be more time consuming than other methods. However, pain and irritation caused by some drugs can be avoided by using the intravenous route. Also, more reliable treatment can be given as more accurate doses can be quickly delivered to target sites (Dougherty and Lister, 2008). The risks of speed shock, anaphylaxis, and phlebitis must also be taken into account (Lavery and Ingram, 2008).

Medicines are commonly administered intravenously via a vascular access device (VAD) (peripheral or central). Use of the intravenous route is not without risks. Key risks include:

- Phlebitis (inflammation of a vein)
- Infiltration (inadvertent administration into the surrounding tissue)
- Haematoma (a collection of blood in the tissue around a vein)
- Air embolism (a bubble in the vein breaking the blood flow)
- Speed shock (fast injection leading to concentration of the injected drug in blood-rich organs, causing toxicity)

- Fluid overload (when the blood vessels contain more fluid than the heart can effectively circulate)
- Septicaemia (blood poisoning, usually due to infection).

(Royal College of Nursing, 2007)

Intrathecal and epidural routes

To explain the need for these routes, we must consider the blood–brain barrier. To protect the brain from infection, much of it lies within a barrier made up of fatty (lipid) membrane with tight junctions between the cells. Bacteria are unable to squeeze through, though some viruses can do so. Similarly, large molecules cannot generally penetrate the brain, which protects it from a range of toxins.

Unfortunately, this protective barrier also prevents the entry of most medication. To be able to pass through the cell barrier, medicines need to be very soluble in lipids (see Table 4.1). Since blood is largely composed of water, lipophilic (lipid-loving) chemicals will leave the blood and enter the lipid membranes when they come into contact with them. It is difficult to deliver large amounts of medication to the brain in this way, although when the brain surfaces are inflamed they become more porous.

The best way to deliver medication to the brain is to bypass the blood–brain barrier by injecting inside it using a catheter introduced into the intrathecal or epidural space. The intrathecal space contains the cerebro-spinal fluid and spinal cord, whereas the epidural space is the narrow sleeve like area outside the

Table 4.1 Lipophilic and hydrophilic drugs.

Lipid soluble drugs (lipophilic drugs)	Water soluble drugs (hydrophilic drugs)
Most drugs are lipophilic which means that they have a liking for fat. Most cell membranes have a fatty layer that makes the movement of other fats into the cell possible. Lipophilic drugs are therefore easily transported by absorption across most cell membranes.	Fat repels water. Hydrophilic drugs, have a liking for water and are repelled by most cell membranes so hydrophilic drugs are not easily transported by passive diffusion into most cells.
The placental barrier is lipophilic which means that most drugs cross this natural barrier and pass into the fetus to a greater or lesser degree.	Despite this, special mechanisms can actively transport hydrophilic drugs into the brain e.g. levodopa (Pardridge, 1998; Alavijeh et al, 2005)

dura mater. Analgesia, given in this way, is absorbed into the spinal cord or nearby nerves and blocks the transmission of pain impulses.

Specially prepared drugs are used for these routes and dosages are usually much smaller than for intramuscular or intravenous injection (Dougherty and Lister, 2008).

Topical or transdermal

This route generally allows local absorption of the drug, via the epidermis which is the outer layer of the skin, and, in this way, reduces the side effects on the body as a whole. However, with transdermal patches the drug is absorbed through the skin and into the blood capillaries. It will then enter the systemic circulation and, therefore, potential systemic side effects cannot be eliminated.

Transdermal delivery provides a relatively constant rate of absorption over a specified time. Some patches can be left in situ for several days before requiring replacement, and they are therefore popular for pain relief in palliative care, or nicotine replacement when patients are trying to stop smoking. However, the rate of absorption can be affected by body temperature (Lilley et al, 2007). Medication delivered using this route is often more costly that an oral preparation and can cause irritation to the skin. Some of these patches are transparent and it is therefore good practice to note on the patient's medication chart where the patch was placed so it can be readily found by colleagues when they need to remove it.

Creams, lotions, ointments, and pastes

There is confusion about the difference between these terms.

Creams are water-based and water-miscible (they can be mixed with water). When applied to dry skin, they release water into the epidermis. Creams such as aqueous cream have very high water content for this purpose.

The process of making a cream is very similar to making a batter in the kitchen with eggs, milk, and flour. While fats or oils and water will not normally mix, the lecithin in the egg yolk acts as an emulsifier and allows tiny stable droplets of oil to remain suspended in the watery part of the milk. Flour is added to thicken the mixture. If oils or fats are to be incorporated in creams, they have to be emulsified first by mixing them with something that will break them into these tiny stable droplets. Most lotions can be regarded as diluted creams, because they are oil-in-water emulsions.

Ointments are prepared in a greasy base. Applied to the epidermis they prevent the release of moisture. When the skin is very dry, ointments are preferred to creams. They are more likely to penetrate dry skin, and they reduce water loss from it, but some patients will not tolerate them because they leave a greasy layer on the skin which may be inconvenient or uncomfortable. Ointments have the added advantage that they are less readily removed when washing, and they are therefore particularly useful for treating hands which may be in water many times a day, whereas creams might need to be reapplied after washing. Water-soluble medications must be emulsified before adding to an ointment. Made in the dispensary, ointments require a little more skill than making creams. Making an ointment is very similar to preparing mayonnaise, which is also a water-in-oil emulsion. Some lotions are water-in-oil emulsions and could therefore be viewed as diluted ointments.

Pastes are thick topical applications with a high solid content. They may be used to draw out the contents of boils or carbuncles by osmosis. The liquid contents of the boil are pulled into the thick paste, encouraging the boil to discharge. They are much less commonly used today than formerly, since we discourage lancing or drawing boils as a matter of course.

Creams and ointments can be easy for patients to apply themselves, although ointments may be less well tolerated as they tend to be greasy. Clear information about how to measure and apply topical medication is vital to ensure its effectiveness and the patient's safety. This is especially important for topical corticosteroids (Downie et al, 2008).

A useful measuring technique that is most often used for topical application is the fingertip unit (FTU), which is the amount of cream or ointment expressed from a tube with a 5 mm diameter nozzle, applied from

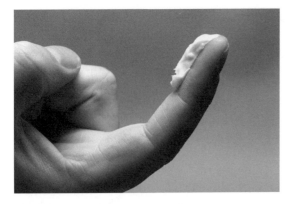

Figure 4.5 A fingertip unit
© Mark Thomas/Science Photo Library

the distal skin-crease to the tip of the index finger. See Figure 4.5.

Once you have established what a fingertip unit looks like you need to know how many to apply depending on the area to be treated. A good guide is one FTU is enough to treat an area of skin twice the size of the flat of an adult's hand with the fingers together. Based on this Table 4.2 gives a guide for application to various body parts and helps to estimate the amount required in adults.

It is vital when applying topical medicines to children that adjustments need to be made to the amounts required for adults. If you continue with an FTU measured on an adult finger, one FTU is used to treat an area of skin on a child equivalent to twice the size of the flat of an adult's hand with the fingers together; then you can use your own (adult) hand to establish the amount of the child's skin that requires treatment and therefore the number of fingertip units you need to use.

It is good practice not to allow topical medicaments (those that are applied rather than taken) to touch your skin. When large volumes are to be applied, impermeable gloves should be worn. For smaller volumes, spatulas are usually available. If creams or ointments are likely to be applied to a particularly hairy area for more than a day or two, it may be helpful to shave the area so that the skin is accessible. When informing patients about how to apply topical medications themselves, be clear about the need for them to wash their hands thoroughly if applying with ungloved hands.

Box 4.3 Shaving

> A disposable razor is more commonly used than an electric razor, partly for reasons of hygiene. With skilled use, a bladed razor will give better results than an electric razor, but it also removes cells from the outer layer of skin. This may be sufficient to increase the absorption of medicines applied to the shaved skin, so it is important to disturb the outer skin layer as little as possible during shaving.

Eye drops and ointments

While prevention of infection is necessary when administering medicines by any route, it is especially important with eyes, as they are particularly susceptible to

Table 4.2 Application of required fingertip units per body part in adults. (Adapted from information by NHS Evidence.)

Area to be treated	Approximate size	FTUs
A hand and fingers (front and back)	About 2 adult hands	One
Front of chest and abdomen	About 14 adult hands	Seven
Back and buttocks	About 14 adult hands	Seven
Face and neck	About 5 adult hands	Two and a half
An entire arm and hand	About 8 adult hands	Four
An entire leg and foot	About 16 adult hands	Eight

FTU, fingertip unit.

infection (Baillie, 2005). This point must be emphasized to patients, as well as the risk of cross infection should only one eye need treatment. Remember that it can be difficult for patients to self-administer eye drops.

The risk of allergy or unpleasant reactions means that many eye preparations contain no preservative or relatively weak antiseptics, and are therefore at risk of becoming contaminated. To minimize this risk, it is good practice to keep separate bottles for each eye if the eyes are already infected, so as not to transfer the infection from the infected eye to the other eye. In addition, the drops are usually kept in a refrigerator between uses. This slows bacterial growth so that if bacteria manage to enter the bottle, they are less likely to multiply. Even so, eye drops should be discarded 28 days after being opened.

Eye ointments, having a base which contains very little water, are not good environments for bacterial growth. However, because the nozzle of the tube may contact an infected eye the same principles apply—keep tubes separate if there is infection and dispose of any unused eye ointment after 28 days.

Summary

This chapter has discussed the many routes for administration of medicines; acknowledging that the oral route is the most commonly used. Nurses need to consider the advantages and disadvantages of using different routes and these have been explored. The form in which medicines are presented and how this might impact on the administration has also been discussed. Ensuring a sound understanding of the formulation of medicines and the variety of routes that can be used will help nurses administer them in a safe and effective manner.

References

Alavijeh MS, Chishty M, Qaiser MZ, and Palmer AM, (2005) Drug Metabolism and Pharmacokinetics, the Blood-Brain Barrier, and Central Nervous System Drug Discovery, *NeuroRx*, 2; 554–571.

Baillie L (2005) *Developing Practical Nursing Skills* 2nd ed. London: Hodder Arnold.

BNF see Joint Formulary Committee.

Diggle L (2007) Injection technique for immunisation, *Practice Nurse*, 33; 34–37.

Dougherty L and Lister S (eds) (2008), *The Royal Marsden Hospital Manual of Clinical Nursing Procedures.* Oxford: Wiley-Blackwell.

Downie G, Mackenzie J, and Williams A (2008), *Pharmacology and Medicines Management for Nurses.* London: Churchill Livingstone.

Glasper A, McEwing G, and Richardson J (2009), *FoundationSkills for Caring.* Basingstoke: Palgrave Macmillan.

Hunter J (2007), Intramuscular injection techniques. *Nursing Standard.* 22(24); 35–40.

Joint Formulary Committee (2012), *British National Formulary* (64th ed). London: BMJ Group and Pharmaceutical Press.

Lavery I, and Ingram P (2008), Safe practice in intravenous medicines administration. *Nursing Standard* 22(46); 44–47.

Lilley L, Harrington S, and Snyder J (2007), *Pharmacology and the Nursing Process.* St Louis, Mosby.

McGavock H (2004), *How drugs work.* Abingdon: Radcliffe Medical Press.

NMC (2008a), *Standards for Medicines Management.* London: NMC.

NMC (2008b), *The Code: Standards of Conduct, Performance and Ethics for Nurses and Midwives.* London: NMC.

Pardridge W A (1998), CNS Drug Design Based on Principles of Blood–Brain Barrier Transport, *J. Neurochem*, 70; 1781–1792.

Pegram A, Bloomfield J, and Jones A (2008), Safe use of rectal suppositories and enemas with adult patients. *Nursing Standard*, 22(38); 38–40.

Perry AG, and Potter PA (2004), *Clinical nursing skills and techniques* (5th ed). St. Louis: Mosby.

Royal College of Nursing (2007), *Standards for Infusion therapy.* London: RCN.

Scott W and McGrath D (2008), *Nursing Pharmacology made incredibly easy.* London: Lippincott Williams and Wilkins.

Trounce J (2000), *Clinical Pharmacology.* London: Churchill Livingstone.

van den Bernt P, Cusell M, Overbeeke P, Trommelen M, van Dooren D, Ophorst W et al (2006), Quality improvement of oral medication administration in patients with enteral feeding tubes. *Quality Safety Health Care,* 15; 44–47.

Workman B (1999), Safe injection techniques. *Nursing Standard,* 13(39); 47–52.

5 Groups at Special Risk of Adverse Effects

CHAPTER CONTENTS

- Groups of patients who are at special risk
- Circumstances that might pose a risk to patients
- The older patient
- Medicines and patients who have hepatic impairment
- Medicines and patients who have renal impairment

- Medicines and the pregnant woman
- Medicines and women who are breastfeeding
- Medicines and children
- Medicines and patients with cognitive impairment and learning disability
- Polypharmacy: the nurse and the patient
- Summary

LEARNING OUTCOMES

In Chapters 3 and 4 the general principles of pharmacokinetics and pharmacodynamics were addressed. This chapter builds on these principles and looks at specific groups and situations.

After reading this chapter you should be able to:

- Identify groups of patients at extra risk of interactions, explain why, and relate this to nursing practice.
- Identify groups of patients at more risk of adverse events from medications, explain why, and relate this to nursing practice.
- Understand why some patients might be at higher risk and how this might be managed.

Groups of patients who are at special risk

This chapter will look at a range of patients from the perspective of the nurse administering medicines. Whilst care must be taken when administering medication to any patient, there are groups of patients where the risk of problems occurring as a result of having to take medication are higher and it is therefore even more important to be vigilant. For some patients the treatment will have to be altered to reduce risk. While this is not the responsibility of the student nurse it is their responsibility to be vigilant to changes in the patient and to report this to trained staff.

Circumstances that might pose a risk to patients

There are some circumstances in which the risk to patients is always higher because the treatment they are receiving carries more risk. For example, patients undergoing cancer chemotherapy are receiving drugs which tend to be highly toxic. While the risk of some degree of harm is high, this is justified by the great benefit that patients can derive. However, it is vital that every effort is made to reduce risk. Similarly there are features of care in acute settings such as operating theatres and intensive care units that could increase the risk to patients (Neale et al, 2001). Staff may be under acute pressure, so it becomes harder to follow all the steps in a routine.

Reflection point

> Reflect on the experiences you might have had when working in acute clinical areas where staff have been under pressure when giving medicines.

The best protection for patients is adherence to good procedures, policies, and protocols. Medicines should be stored in a standard layout so they can be quickly found when needed. All organizations should have a medicines policy that indicates procedure for staff. Departments will have procedures for recording the medicines that are used; all nurses need to be familiar with these and understand their role. (Exercise 5.1 will help you to do this.)

When you are asked to check the identity of a medicine take your time. Medicines should never be drawn up in advance and left in unlabelled syringes. If medicines need to be mixed within a syringe, or saline or water has to be added to dilute them, all the ingredients should be to hand before anything is drawn up to prevent the undiluted drug being given accidentally. It is everybody's responsibility to challenge practice that may present risk to the patient (NMC, 2010).

Generic and branded drugs

It is important for the nurse to familiarize themselves with the name and details of all of the drugs that

Exercise 5.1

> - When you are next in practice ask to see the medicines policy. This is often located on the staff intranet.
> - From the medicines policy, identify the roles and responsibilities of the trained nurse in relation to the administration of medicines to patients.
> - Make a list of the important points in the medicines policy that relate to the role of the trained nurse
>
> Discuss these with your mentor—this may be used as evidence to demonstrate your progression.

their patient might be taking. You might find it useful to keep a notebook with these in. Most drugs are prescribed under what is known as their generic name. For example the generic name for Lasix (a diuretic) is furosemide. Lasix is the brand name that is used by the drug company who make it (BNF, 2012). Generally the branded drug is more expensive than the generic and prescribers are encouraged, where possible, to prescribe generically as this can save money. However, it is important for all nurses to note that not all drugs should be prescribed in their generic form. Some medicines are available in brands with slightly different absorption profiles which lead to differences in the blood levels achieved. For this reason the *BNF* suggests that in some circumstances the brand to be used should be specified. (BNF, 2012).

The cartoon in Figure 5.1 suggests that the lady who is asking for the medicine believes (possibly) that the generic medicine might be of inferior quality compared with the brand medicine. This is not the case and nurses need to be aware that patients might ask why they are being given a different version of their usual medicine. They may be thinking that their medicine has been changed and might not be as effective. There is also a potential risk that patients could be prescribed both the generic and branded version of the same medicine.

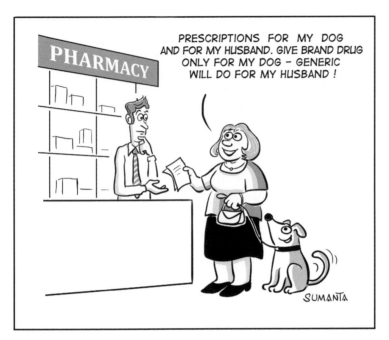

Figure 5.1 Generic versus brand name drugs.
Courtesy of Sumanta Baruah (www.cartooncosmos.com)

Reflection point

- Have you cared for a patient who needed a branded medicine?
- What was the medicine?
- Read about it in the *BNF*
- Why did the patient need that medicine?
- What would the nurse need to be aware of when caring for a patient who is taking this medicine?

The older patient

Chapters 3 and 4 gave an introduction to pharmacokinetics and pharmacodynamics and it will be useful to refer back to these when reading onwards. The proportion of the UK population over 60 was 22.1% in 2008; this is projected to rise to 28.8% by 2033. See the national population projections table 3.2 at: **http://www.ons.gov.uk/ons/rel/pop-estimate/population-estimates-for-uk--england-and-wales--scotland-and-northern-ireland/population-density-tables-1981-to-2010/index.html**.

We need to be aware that nurses will be caring for increasing numbers of older people. There are suggestions for further reading at the end of this chapter.

Older people who are patients generally carry more risk than others for two reasons:

1 They tend to have a number of long-term conditions, so they generally need more treatment, and therefore are at more risk from polypharmacy.

2 Even if they do not need more medicines, their ability to tolerate some medicines may be reduced, even though they may have been taking them for a long time (Hilmer, 2008).

For example, glibenclamide is used in patients with diabetes in order to lower their blood sugar (BNF, 2012). It has the advantage that it is long-acting, so patients usually only need to take it once a day. However, with increasing age their ability to metabolize glibenclamide declines (BNF, 2012). The result is that the drug's duration of action is extended, and this can lead to hypoglycaemia—low blood sugar—resulting in coma or even death (Tessier et al, 1994). These patients may be very reluctant to have their treatment changed at 75 or 80 years of age, when they have been using a certain medicine for twenty years or more, but their risk of harm has increased and action must be taken to protect them.

How ageing affects the processing of drugs

In order to minimize the risk of adverse reactions and interactions, an understanding of the ageing process is essential, remembering always that the individual in front of us may be an exception to the general ageing pattern. While generally a person's body will deteriorate with age and this will affect how the body processes the medicine and also the effect the medicine has on the body, each person is an individual and their rate of change will depend on many complex variables. The nurse must be aware that each patient is unique and as such might react in a less predictable fashion. There is a suggestion at the end of this chapter for further reading about the ageing process.

Changes in pharmacokinetics

Pharmacokinetics can be defined as the effect the body has on the drug, and can be divided into four phases:

- Absorption
- Distribution
- Metabolism
- Elimination.

(You may wish to refresh your understanding by revisiting Chapter 3.)

Whilst this section focuses on the pharmacokinetics of oral drugs, similar considerations apply to drugs given by other routes. For example, older patients may experience skin thinning, reduced tissue perfusion, and a changed body fat percentage which may affect absorption from subcutaneous injections and transdermal patches, and reduced muscle mass may affect the activity of intramuscular injections (Turnheim, 2003).

Absorption

Absorption of orally administered drugs depends on several key factors. One which is often overlooked is a patient's inability to chew. Nurses are in an ideal position to assess dental health and the possibility of poorly fitting dentures. Also, 25% of older people

Exercise 5.2

> Many older people take calcium tablets. These must be chewed before swallowing, but the tablets are large and hard, so some older people cannot effectively chew them. As a nurse, how could you help patients who have difficulty chewing?

produce less saliva, which also inhibits chewing and reduces absorption through the buccal mucosa (Vissink et al, 1996).

When the medicine reaches the patient's stomach decreased gastric acid production, which occurs in many as part of the ageing process, slows the dissolution of tablets. The rhythmic contraction of the intestines (peristalsis) becomes weaker with ageing, because the autonomic nervous system that controls it becomes less reactive. The result is that the patient's gastric emptying lime is increased, which may also influence the degree of absorption (Mangoni and Jackson, 2004). In this case, absorption is more likely to be increased, because the medicine will be in contact with the intestinal mucosa for longer.

However, in the older patient, the mucosa is likely to be less efficient. Absorption depends upon the surface area. In younger people the mucosa has many tiny folds to increase the area, but as we age epithelial atrophy reduces the surface area for absorption. The mucosa becomes flatter and absorbs less. Decreased motility may compensate for this by prolonging contact between the drug and the mucosa, which explains why constipated patients may absorb more of some medicines (Gidal, 2006).

Distribution

Several factors affect distribution, but it is largely dependent on the efficiency of the cardiovascular system. In older people, the heart pumps less efficiently and hardening of the arteries causes resistance to blood flow. Reduced cardiac output and increased vascular resistance slows blood flow, leading to decreased perfusion of the liver and kidneys. With a slower supply of drug to these organs the amount that can be processed will be reduced (Armour and Cairns, 2002).

In the older person, plasma protein production may be reduced by 10–20% reducing binding of drugs which bind extensively to albumin (Wallace and Verbeek, 1987; Thompson, 2004). Chronic inflammation as experienced by a proportion of older people may increase the production of α_1-acid glycoprotein leading to increased binding of the drugs in Box 5.1. These changes in plasma protein levels lead to greater variability and unpredictability in protein binding. For some medicines this is unimportant, but for medicines where the fraction that is bound to plasma protein is higher, such as warfarin or phenytoin, this can have serious clinical consequences as a higher proportion of the medicine will be left unbound and therefore free to produce an immediate effect. With reduced protein binding, the risk of displacement of one medicine from protein by another medicine will increase. Again, the patient may have been receiving the same dose of the same medicine for many years without difficulty, but the risk arises as their body systems become less efficient. Nurses may therefore see signs consistent with an apparent overdose in patients receiving normal doses of medicine.

Box 5.1 Examples of medicines which bind extensively to albumin and are used widely for the treatment of conditions in older people:

> Non-steroidal anti-inflammatory drugs (NSAIDs)
> Anticoagulants (particularly warfarin)
> Furosemide
> Phenytoin.
> (Armour and Cairns, 2002).

It is important to assess the patient regularly for nutritional status, dehydration, and body mass index. One example of an assessment tool is the Malnutrition Universal Screening Tool (MUST) available at: **http://www.bapen.org.uk/musttoolkit.html**.

Exercise 5.3

> There are other screening tools in use. Can you think of examples used in your area?

With increasing age, lean body mass decreases while body fat may increase (St-Onge, 2005) and body water is also reduced even in the absence of obvious dehydration. The distribution of medicines stored primarily in either lipids or aqueous body fluids will be affected accordingly, with fat-soluble medicines being more readily stored and the concentration of water soluble medicines increasing. As the patient's stores reach capacity further absorption of medicine will be restricted because in many cases absorption depends on a difference in concentration across a membrane that will not be present if tissues are full. Lipid storage creates a reservoir from which medicines are released as concentration at the site of action decreases. This explains why lipid soluble medicines such as sleeping tablets like benzodiazepines may have a prolonged effect in the older patient. The reduced body water in the older person means that a given dose of a water soluble medicine such as digoxin or gentamicin produces a higher concentration in the plasma. That means that the starting (or 'loading') dose will need to be lower in the older patient, and any increase in dose will be in smaller steps (McGavock, 2010).

Changes in metabolism

To recap from Chapter 3, metabolism is the chemical process by which the body converts medicines into a form suitable for elimination. In the first stage cytochrome enzymes make the medicines more chemically reactive leading to the second stage where the metabolite is joined to a water soluble carrier to remove it (McGavock, 2010).

The generally reduced blood flow to the liver as a result of cardiovascular changes in an older person, results in a reduced first-pass effect. This reduction in first-pass metabolism results in higher levels of free circulating medicine. In addition, cytochrome enzymes are proteins that have to be manufactured in the body. Protein synthesis declines with age, so the cytochrome system in the liver is less active resulting in a slower breakdown of the drug and hence prolonged activity in the body. These changes will result in an increased half-life of the medicine in the older person compared with younger people (McGavock, 2010). Nurses should be aware that either the dose or the frequency of dosing of a medicine may need to vary to allow for this. Not only does the cytochrome system slow down but the conjugation system also slows leading to more partially metabolized drug which may be active in the body for a longer period. This is significant in the case of prodrugs where the metabolite is an active compound. An example is seen with opiate analgesics where the metabolized products are also active drugs.

Elimination

Although there is always an exception to the rule, reduced cardiovascular blood flow in the older person restricts the efficiency of the kidneys. The majority of elimination takes place in the kidney and its rate depends on the difference in concentration of the medicine at the glomerulus. Even in the absence of obvious kidney disease, the number of glomeruli will fall by about a third in the older person and active processes in the kidney such as secretion and reabsorption are diminished Armour and Cairns (2002). Together, these changes lead to impaired renal function which results in higher levels of medicine in the plasma.

A standard monitoring test for kidney function is serum creatinine. This creatinine is produced from the breakdown of our muscles, and during most of our life this proceeds at a constant rate. The kidneys remove the creatinine produced, so measuring the creatinine in the blood gives us a simple measure of kidney efficiency. However, as a result of declining muscle mass, we produce less creatinine as we age, so the serum creatinine in the older person may appear normal despite significant renal impairment (Lindeman, 1992). This explains why changes in medicines may be necessary despite apparently normal creatinine levels. A fuller explanation can be found in Appendix 3 of the latest edition of the *British National Formulary*.

Summary of pharmacokinetic changes that may affect older patients

Medicines may accumulate in older people because:

- They are absorbed differently
- They are distributed to different tissues or in different proportions between tissues

- Their metabolism is less efficient
- Their elimination is reduced.

Pharmacodynamic changes

Pharmacodynamics can be defined as the interaction between the drug and the receptors at the site of action in the body. Ageing affects the pharmacodynamic process in several ways. As a result of decreased protein synthesis the numbers of receptors tend to decrease in the older person (McGavock, 2010). Secondly, the affinity of the drug for the receptor depends on the fit between the drug and the receptor which may change because the receptors produced are structurally deficient—they may be badly made so the fit of the drug is not as good—due to the general ageing process. See: **http://www.nottingham.ac.uk/nursing/sonet/rlos/bioproc/lock_and key/2.html** for an animation showing the lock and key hypothesis of drug-receptor interaction.

Finally, the target organ might not respond to the stimulus as effectively as it would in younger people (McGavock, 2010).

Adverse drug reactions in older people

The causes of adverse drug reactions (ADRs) in older people comprise a complex picture (Gurwitz and Avorn, 1991). Type A reactions are dose related and for the reasons already given older people may have higher blood levels for the same dose and are therefore more prone to these reactions. Caution needs to be exercised particularly when prescribing drugs with a narrow therapeutic range such as digoxin and theophylline (McGavock, 2010).

In younger people a potential ADR may be compensated for by another body mechanism. In older people, this compensating mechanism may be absent or inadequate. For example, lisinopril can cause postural hypotension (BNF, 2012), which may be particularly marked in older people, whose blood vessels are not as elastic, therefore the reflex vasoconstriction that occurs in younger people might not be present.

Medicines and patients who have hepatic impairment

Patients of all ages can have liver impairment; however, it becomes increasingly common with age. The liver is largely responsible for the metabolism of many medicines. If its functioning is impaired, this will have a major effect on the extent to which medicines can be metabolized and may require the patient's treatment to be changed. However, liver function tests do not accurately describe the capacity of an individual to metabolize medicines. Since the liver is a large organ with plenty of spare capacity, impairment has to be quite severe before metabolism is seriously affected.

Liver impairment can cause alterations in many factors such as intestinal absorption, plasma protein binding, hepatic blood flow, excretion via bile, and enterohepatic circulation. Given this variety and complexity of effects, it is difficult to predict levels and effects for an individual drug and patient. The type and severity of liver impairment does not predict these either, so no general rules are available for adjusting medicinal dosage in patients with liver disease (Porth et al, 2010).

Impairment of hepatic metabolism means increased half-lives for many drugs. Reduced hepatic blood flow means that there will also be a reduced first-pass effect. Since metabolism will be slower, the levels of drugs in the circulation will tend to rise, active metabolites will be increased, and their effects will last longer (McGavock, 2010).

In severe liver disease, plasma proteins are reduced. As a result the protein-bound fraction of medicine may fall, leaving more medicine free in the circulation, causing an enhanced effect and more toxicity. Medicines which are highly protein-bound such as phenytoin (an anticonvulsant), prednisolone (a steroid), and warfarin (an anticoagulant) are most likely to be affected.

Medicines that cause dose-related toxicity may do so at a lower dose than usual. Unpredictable or idiosyncratic adverse reactions may be more common in patients with hepatic impairment.

For more information about the liver see Further Reading.

Medicines and patients who have renal impairment

As for hepatic disease, older patients are also likely to have renal insufficiency. It is the role of the nurse to ensure a thorough assessment of the patient. Reduced renal function can cause:

• Toxicity due to failure to excrete a drug or its metabolites,

• Increased patient sensitivity to some medicines even if elimination is unimpaired,

• Reduced patient toleration of side-effects (in renal failure),

• Reduced clinical effectiveness of some medicines.

Many problems for patients can be avoided by reducing the dose or using alternative medication.

It will not normally be the duty of a nurse to adjust doses in patients with kidney or liver failure. However, it is important that nurses caring for such patients are particularly alert to any adverse effects.

For more information about the kidney see Further Reading.

Medicines and the pregnant woman

Although women who are pregnant receive their maternity care mainly from the midwife it is important to remember that they might have medical conditions for which they need medical treatment and nursing care and as such they may need to take medicine. Pregnant women, in the same way as any other group of patients, might also be prescribed medicines that they are taking at home or be self-treating with medicines that they have obtained over the counter (OTC) or from pharmacists (P medicines). Therefore it is important that nurses have some knowledge of the role of the nurse in relation to medicines management and pregnant women.

Medicines can be harmful to the fetus at any time during pregnancy, and it is therefore normal practice only to offer them when the benefit to the mother outweighs the risk to the baby. During the first trimester (three months) of pregnancy, the baby's limbs and organs are being formed. There is therefore a potential risk of malformation, especially between the third and eleventh week of pregnancy. For this reason we will try to avoid all except the most essential medication. The *BNF* notes a small number of medicines which have not been shown to be harmful, but the best advice is never to give any medicine that has not been prescribed by a doctor or other trained prescriber, however innocuous it may seem.

In the second and third trimesters the baby grows in size and the tissues develop. Medicines given during this time are unlikely to cause physical malformations, but may be toxic to growing organs. In addition, medicines given to women in the stages of late pregnancy may have an adverse effect on labour. For example salbutamol, a β-agonist which is given to people with asthma, also has the effect of slowing or stopping contractions of the uterus, thereby prolonging a woman's labour.

The *BNF* (2012) does not have clear advice on the suitability of all medicines in pregnancy. In general, it notes those which are known to be harmful and a small number where experience suggests they are not likely to cause harm, but for the vast majority there is insufficient evidence to form a view. Of course, it would be highly unethical to give medicines to pregnant women to see if they damaged their babies.

One problem that cannot be avoided is that damage may be done before women realize that they are pregnant. It is therefore customary to be cautious before prescribing for or giving medicines to women of childbearing age and sometimes they will be counselled to take contraceptive precautions while they are taking particular medicines that may harm a fetus. If you become aware that a woman is pregnant, but the person who is helping her to manage her medication did not know this, it is important that her treatment is promptly reviewed to see if any medicines must be stopped. It is the responsibility of the nurse to act, at all times, in the best interest of the patient (NMC, 2008). However, there can sometimes be a conflict between this and the duty of confidentiality (NMC, 2008). For example, if a woman wants the information about her pregnancy kept confidential, the nurse needs to assess

Case study 5.1

> Miss X, who has epilepsy and is taking regular anticonvulsant therapy, is admitted to the Emergency Department having had a fit. She discloses to you that she is 8 weeks pregnant. She does not want the doctor to know as she has not yet told her boyfriend, who is on his way to collect her.
>
> Consider this and discuss with your mentor how you might manage this situation.

the balance of risks to mother and baby and discuss these with the mother (see Case study 5.1).

Medicines and women who are breastfeeding

Although women who are breastfeeding are cared for in the early stages by the midwife, this care stops after the first month of the child's life. It is important to remember that women who are breastfeeding might have medical conditions for which they need to take medicine and also that they might be taking contraception in the form of progesterone, either orally or as an implant. Women who are breastfeeding, in the same way as any other group of patients might also be self-treating with medicines that they have obtained over the counter or from pharmacists.

Medicines may produce a range of problems in breastfeeding:

- Medicines in breast milk may harm the infant
- They may inhibit lactation in the mother
- They may not be harmful, but their presence in the milk may stop baby wanting to feed (e.g. they may give the milk a bad taste).

Again, the *BNF* (2012) contains information about the use of medicines in breastfeeding. As for women who are pregnant, there are some medicines known to be harmful to the baby, some of which are believed not to be harmful (or present in such small quantities that they are unlikely to be harmful), and others for which information is lacking. However, since the milk can be intercepted and its drug content can be checked, it is easier to determine the safety of medicines in breastfeeding than in pregnancy. Sometimes a medicine's known chemical properties allow us to predict that it will not pass into breast milk.

Generally, medicines that are poorly absorbed or have a high first-pass metabolism are less likely to be problematical to the feeding baby during breastfeeding. For example, the antibiotic gentamicin is highly hydrophilic and is very poorly absorbed when administered orally. Gentamicin is therefore unlikely to pass into breast milk in quantities that could be damaging to a baby. Medicines which consist of very large molecules such as insulin are unlikely to pass into breast milk; those which are lipid soluble are more likely to do so than those which are water soluble.

A small number of medicines concentrate in breast milk. One such medicine is iodine. At one time women who suffered perineal damage during labour might have iodine-releasing antiseptic dressings applied. On rare occasions sufficient iodine was absorbed to turn the milk orange; this is no longer done. If you are asked to apply an antiseptic dressing to a breastfeeding mother with a large raw area, it is best to ask for advice on a suitable product from a senior colleague.

Some sleeping tablets will inhibit the baby's sucking reflex, interfering with their feeding, while a few may alter the flavour of the milk. Pseudoephedrine, which is a decongestant found in some cough and cold cures, does not enter milk in quantities that should cause harm, but some babies dislike its bitter taste and seem to be very sensitive to it. Although the main ingredient may not enter milk in sufficient quantities to cause harm, remember that the other ingredients such as flavourings and colourings may still pass and affect the baby's willingness to accept the milk.

Even though the concentrations of a medicine may seem to be too low to cause harm, it must not be forgotten that medicines in breast milk may cause hypersensitivity reactions in the infant.

Medicines and children

The nursing care of the sick child and the support of their family falls within the competency domain of the registered children's nurse. If your focus is nursing children or you are training to become a registered children's nurse then it is important to be aware of the issues that relate to managing medicines for children and for their families. However, as children are generally cared for as part of a wider family it is a good idea for all registered nurses and nurses in training in any field of practice to have an awareness of some of the key points that are related to medication management for children. Remember that you must only ever provide care and advice if you are competent to do so and if it falls within your area of practice; so always seek advice if you are not sure (NMC, 2008). Remember that decisions regarding children must be made in partnership with the parents or legal guardians who may be experts in their child's care (Children Act, 1989). Where possible it is important also to involve the child in such decision making. Doses for children should be based on advice from standard texts such as the *British National Formulary for Children* (BNFC, 2012–2013).

Generally medicines which have a licence or marketing authorization granted by the Medicines and Healthcare Products Regulatory Agency (MHRA) should always be used in preference to unlicensed ones (see Chapter 1). Unfortunately very few drugs are licensed for use in children; one study found that barely half the drugs used on hospital paediatric wards were licensed for their use. (Conroy et al, 2000). Reasons might be:

- The cost of research necessary to obtain a licence. If doctors are going to prescribe the product anyway, it is obvious why the manufacturers might not bother.

- Research in adults is often done using informed volunteers who give their consent. Small children are generally unable to consent to interventions, and their parents' right to do so is dependent on the proposed action being in the child's best interest (The Children Act, 1989). It is difficult to prove that a new medicine is in the child's best interest when information on its safety is very limited but gathering this data is a key reason for wanting to do the research. It may therefore be unethical to do some of the work that we would ideally wish to do.

European regulations now address this problem through a carrot and stick approach. Manufacturers applying for a licence for a new medicine have to put forward a paediatric investigation plan (PIP) which will gather at least some basic information on the use of their medicine in children. The process is described at: **http://www.ema.europa.eu/ema/index.jsp?curl=pages/regulation/q_and_a/q_and_a_detail_000015.jsp&mid=WC0b01ac0580025b8e**.

In exchange for doing this, their patent is effectively extended a little, giving them some extra time to recoup the costs before their drug can be copied by others. When the work in the PIP has been completed, the drug may be awarded a PUMA—a paediatric use marketing authorization. This is achieved via a special abbreviated procedure described at: **http://www.ema.europa.eu/docs/en_GB/document_library/Other/2011/09/WC500112071.pdf**.

The reduced licensing programme and the continuing need to use some unlicensed products places a duty on all of us to be particularly vigilant in watching for evidence of medicine-induced harm in children. All suspected adverse effects should be reported, however trivial. Anyone can report these via the yellow card scheme (see Chapter 2 for details) but in most hospitals nurses are encouraged to seek the advice of a senior colleague before making a report. This has the added advantage of reducing the risk of double counting due to two people on a ward making reports on the same incident.

Many firms prepare special formulations of their medicines for use in children. However, it is important not to assume that a liquid medicine is always suitable for a child. It is also important to remember that the adverse events experienced by children may not be related to the active ingredient in a medicine. Nurses should be aware that the excipients (items added to the medicine to prepare it in a form that can be taken) may themselves cause adverse reactions, especially in children, who may be sensitive to flavourings and preservatives. Occasionally, concerned parents will ask whether a medicine can be prepared 'without E numbers'. It must be remembered that some 'E numbers' are perfectly safe or natural products. For example, E414 is gum arabic; E300 is vitamin C; E330 is citric acid. Often the parents mean that they want medicines without colours or preservatives. Modern practice is for manufacturers only to include these items if they think they are needed. Antibiotic mixtures are commonly sugar-free and many are now colour-free, but colours may be added to give a consistent appearance to a natural product or to disguise an unappetising look. For example, the antihistamine chlorphenamine produces a muddy-coloured liquid, so makers will often add a yellow or orange colour. Nurses who are working with children and their families must be aware that although it is important always to take the views and wishes of parents into account it is not always possible to meet them without compromising the efficacy of the treatment. Flavourings may improve adherence, because children are less willing than adults to take something that tastes unpleasant. This can itself be a safety feature. Solutions of methadone, a medicine used in the treatment of opiate addiction, do not taste pleasant. While the taste of methadone is hard to disguise anyway, the manufacturers do not do so partly so that children who might attempt to drink it will be put off by the bitter taste.

Within the limitations of their understanding, children must be given an explanation of their treatment and some involvement in setting the goals for that treatment. This requires the nurse to assess the level of understanding that a child has and use this assessment to tailor the information given to explain what their medicine is intended to do and how it must be used to best effect. The child may be able to point to factors impeding good adherence; for example, there may be a school rule that prevents them carrying medicines, or they may have lunch at different times during the school week, making their insulin dosing more difficult.

Differences in paediatric pharmacokinetics

Absorption

In babies, gastric emptying time is prolonged and only approaches adult values at around six months of age. In older infants, intestinal hurry may occur, in which the involuntary movements of the intestines are accelerated, often producing diarrhoea because the contents are not in contact with the gut mucosa long enough to resorb as much water as usual. Either of these factors may affect the proportion of an oral dose that the child absorbs or the speed with which it can absorb a medicine.

In addition, a child's gastric acid output does not reach adult values until the second year of life, so the pH level in the stomach is higher. Unionized medicines—those with neither a positive nor a negative charge—are more readily absorbed through the young child's intestinal lining. Given the higher pH of the child's stomach, some medicines will not ionize to the same degree in children as they would in adults. Some medicines do not ionize to a large extent, so the effect is minimal, but others are very readily ionized. As a result it is possible that the reduced stomach acid will allow some medicines to be more readily absorbed in small children.

Distribution

As a percentage of total weight, the total body water and extracellular fluid volume decrease with increasing age, so neonates need higher doses of water soluble medicines on a mg/kg basis than adults, because their bodies contain more water per kilogram than adults' bodies do.

Neonates have low levels of albumin and globulins and therefore a reduced plasma protein binding capacity. High levels of bilirubin in the circulation of neonates may displace medicines from albumin. With less protein binding there is more of the free drug, so doses may have to be decreased to avoid overdose.

Metabolism

Enzyme systems mature at different times. They may be absent at birth, or much less effective. Children may also have different metabolic pathways for some medicines. Generally, these immature or variant enzyme systems mean that the half-life of many medicines is likely to be doubled in children compared with adults (Berlin, 2009). These variations in enzyme systems mean that the first phase of metabolism is reduced in neonates,

but increases progressively during the first six months of life. In early childhood it may exceed adult rates for some medicines, but then slows to adult rates by the child's teenage years.

Compared with adults, children may require more frequent dosing or higher doses on a mg/kg basis. This is particularly true in children under 12 years of age, where the higher metabolic rate enables them to clear medicines more quickly than adults, and hence shorten the medicine's half-life. Logically, the correct way to respond to changes in half-life is to change the dosing interval, because the dosing interval should depend on the half-life; both are measured in units of time, after all. However, the complications of patient personalized dosage schedules, especially on hospital wards, mean that we commonly adjust the amount given so that the drug levels stay within the therapeutic range (see Chapter 3 for a definition) for longer.

An added complication is that there is greater variability in the efficiency of metabolism in children of the same age than there is in adults. Moreover, the efficiency of the systems may be different depending on the drugs being given.

Excretion

For most medicines, the excretion rate depends largely on the efficiency of the kidneys. Complete maturation of renal function is not reached until 6–8 months of age at the earliest, and some children may not achieve this until the age of 2 years. It must also be remembered that the relevant date for premature babies may be their expected date of birth, rather than the date that they were born. A baby who is 8 weeks premature will have systems which are much less developed than a child born at full term on the same day.

Kidney efficiency in any person depends on renal plasma flow (the rate at which blood reaches the kidney) and glomerular filtration rate or GFR (the rate at which it is filtered by the kidney). Renal plasma flow is around 12 ml/min at birth and only reaches adult levels of 140 ml/min towards the child's first birthday. Similarly, GFR quickly rises from 2–4 ml/min at birth to 8–20 ml/min within 72 hours, but will take a further 3–5 months to reach adult levels of 120 ml/min. Medicines that are excreted by the kidneys may therefore accumulate. This is particularly important for medicines where the metabolites are active. For example, the painkiller codeine derives most of its activity from its conversion by cytochrome enzymes to morphine. A small child may or may not be able to complete this transformation, but if it can, then it is important that its kidneys should be able to void the morphine produced, or it will accumulate and cause an overdose. For this reason the *BNFC* particularly notes that predicting the correct dose of codeine for small children is especially difficult.

Information giving to parents and children

There are special considerations with respect to giving medicines to children:

- Doses of less than 5 mL should be given from a special oral syringe rather than a spoon to assist in accurate measurement. These syringes are often coloured purple so that they will not be confused with syringes for injections, and they are designed so that a standard needle will not attach. The contents should not be squirted directly down a child's throat. The safest method is to point the syringe into the inside of the cheek to reduce the risk of choking.

- It is best to avoid adding medicines to drinks or feeds. The chief difficulty is that if the child does not take the whole drink, it is difficult to determine the dose that they have received. In addition, there is a risk that interactions will occur, particularly with the protein in the milk, and if the milk is warm, it may affect the stability of the medicine.

- Some products used, especially in hospitals, may not be commercially available, and will have to be obtained from a manufacturer, so it is important that stock levels should be carefully monitored and time allowed to obtain repeat supplies. If a child is being discharged home, it may be necessary to arrange for further supplies to be obtained via the hospital, so the parents or carers must be counselled to allow time for this.

Medicines and patients with cognitive impairment and learning disability

It is important not to generalize about patients with cognitive impairment, mental illnesses, or learning disability and they cannot be included under the same umbrella. This chapter however, highlights patients who are at risk when considering medicines optimization and management. It is important for nurses to be aware that although they may not specialize in either mental health nursing or learning disability, it is likely that they will be faced at some time by patients in non-specialist settings who require general nursing due to comorbidities such as diabetes, heart disease, and thyroid problems to name a few (Smith, 2001; Scott, et al, 2009). However, cognitive impairment does not necessarily lead to physical health problems, nor does it increase the likelihood of adverse effects. The chief concern for nurses is that some patients may be unaware of, or unable to draw our attention to, signs and symptoms that might require a change of treatment.

As with any patient, some will be co-operative with treatment, well-informed about and interested in their condition, and will report adverse effects with accuracy. Others may lack awareness of their condition, or their condition itself may influence their engagement with their treatment. However, it could be that a patient who is suffering hallucinations as a symptom of their cognitive impairment may also be experiencing genuine visual disturbances from their medication, and this highlights the importance of obtaining a thorough history and assessment. It is therefore vital that reports, however they sound, are properly investigated. Where an important side-effect may be anticipated, it is reasonable to ask the patient directly whether they are experiencing it. In some cases, learning disabilities are part of a syndrome which incorporates metabolic changes that might affect the way in which they handle medicines (Smith, 2001; Hafeez, et al, 2007). Safe management of medication rests again on the importance of accurate history taking and assessment.

Chapter 9 will look at the more difficult question of how to promote concordance in patients with cognitive impairment.

For more detailed information the reader is encouraged to refer to more specific texts on psychopharmacology and medication management for mental health (see Further Reading).

Polypharmacy: the nurse and the patient

What is polypharmacy?

A simple definition of polypharmacy is that the patient is concurrently receiving a lot of medicines (NMC, 2010). There is no particular threshold at which we say polypharmacy has begun, but typically we become more concerned when a patient is taking four or more medicines (DH, 2001). Remember that patients might also be self-medicating with medicines—including herbal remedies—that they have bought themselves from the supermarket, the corner shop, or from the pharmacist. When taking a medicines history, these should be enquired about to ensure that you have a complete picture. Over the counter and herbal medicines may cause adverse reactions and interactions. For further information, see: **http://www.cppe.ac. uk/learning/Details.asp?TemplateID=Older-D-02&Format=D&ID=0&EventID=39396**.

Why do nurses need to know?

Nurses need to be aware that polypharmacy is becoming increasingly common as treatments become available for more conditions. In one study it was found that half the population over the age of 60 was receiving five or more medicines. Just under a quarter of these patients received as many as 10 separate medicines, and the highest number was seen in a patient receiving 51 drugs (Hippisley-Cox et al, 2004), see Figure 5.2. This study can be accessed by clicking onto the following link and registering with the site: **http://www.qresearch.org**.

A Dutch study found that 5.5% of patients in general practice over 64 years old using two or more drugs simultaneously suffered adverse effects (Veehof et al, 1999). The prevalence of adverse drug reactions in hospitals remains around 10% of all hospital admissions, although not all of these are due to polypharmacy (Lazarou et al, 1998; Koh et al, 2005). The risk of adverse drug reactions is strongly associated with increasing numbers of drugs taken.

A quick calculation will show why this may be so. If you have two drugs, there is one possible interaction because there is one pairing. (The interaction may also produce more than one adverse effect.) If you have three drugs, A, B, and C, there are three pairings—AB, AC, and BC, and so three (or more) possible interactions. Increasing the number of drugs increases the number of pairings (see Table 5.1).

In algebraic terms, if you have n drugs, the number of pairings is $n (n - 1) / 2$. In fact, the risk is higher than it first appears, because there may also be three-way interactions, though these are unusual. The patient mentioned earlier who was receiving 51 drugs has at least $(51 \times 50) / 2 = 1275$ potential interactions. Obviously,

60+ age group

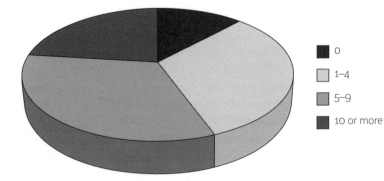

- 0
- 1–4
- 5–9
- 10 or more

Figure 5.2 The number of drugs being taken by patients over 60 years old. Polypharmacy in the elderly, 2004. Reproduced with permission from **http://www.qresearch.org**.

Table 5.1 Number of pairings between different numbers of drugs.

Drugs	Pairings
2	1
3	3
4	6
5	10
6	15
7	21

the greater the number of possible interactions the harder it becomes for the prescriber to examine each risk in detail and predict what will happen. This is why polypharmacy poses a risk to patients.

However, nurses need to be aware that polypharmacy cannot always be avoided. The prevalence of chronic, long-term conditions increases with age, therefore the number of medicines that a patient is likely to need will also increase with age (Hilmer, 2008).

The body will be most challenged by multiple medicines at a time of life when its ability to withstand adverse effects is declining (see section on the older patient earlier in this chapter). In one exercise, doctors were given case notes for a hypothetical 79-year-old woman with chronic obstructive pulmonary disease, type 2 diabetes, osteoporosis, hypertension, and osteoarthritis. Application of evidence-based published guidelines led to recommendations for 12 medications, with high risks of interactions and adverse reactions. These doctors were prescribing what evidence said they should (Boyd et al, 2005).

Some consequences of polypharmacy

Hilmer (2008), notes that the increased risk of adverse reactions is not the only negative consequence of polypharmacy. The more medicines a patient takes, the harder it may be for the nurse to obtain an accurate medication history, without which clinicians lack the information they need for high-quality, informed medicines management and prescribing. If you don't know what a patient has been taking, how do you know what works for that patient? Polypharmacy is a barrier to adherence because of the associated complex medication regimens, increased risk of adverse drug events, and high medication costs. That is, patients are less likely to take their medicines as intended because they find it harder to remember all the instructions that they have been given; they can be put off by side effects or interactions that they may experience; and, if they have to pay prescription charges, the cost may mean that they only request some of their prescribed medications at the pharmacy. Poor adherence by patients to medicines that they have initially agreed to take means that patients will not derive all the benefit they might have done from their medication. There is also a risk that if they are admitted to hospital, where their medicines are administered by others, taking the full dose of medicines that they have not been taking properly before may cause them harm (see Case study 5.2).

Self-assessment

- What is the pathophysiology of congestive heart failure?
- Which medicines are commonly prescribed for congestive heart failure?
- What would you have done if Mrs O had confided in you that she was not taking her medicines but that she did not want you to tell the doctor?
- What is your duty of care in this situation?

Polypharmacy and patients who self–medicate: the role of the nurse

Whilst we have been concentrating here on prescribed medicines, it must be remembered that medicines that patients buy can also interact. One example is that of patients who use indigestion remedies of the white chalky liquid type, such as aluminium hydroxide mixture. This may inhibit the absorption of other drugs, partly because the aluminium forms clumps with the drug particles but also because the reduced acidity of the stomach may slow dissolution of tablets, particularly those with an acid-sensitive

Case study 5.2

Mrs O had congestive heart failure, for which she was prescribed a number of medicines. Her cardiac insufficiency caused the collection of exudate in her lungs. Her GP prescribed a diuretic so that she could expel some of this fluid, but after a couple of episodes of incontinence, Mrs O stopped taking these tablets. (Figure 5.3 is a photograph of Mrs O.)

When her condition worsened, her GP increased the dose, but Mrs O did not tell him that she was not taking the diuretics because she thought he would be cross with her. Mrs O became very poorly and was admitted to hospital. The consultant there saw from her notes that she had been prescribed 80 mg furosemide, a diuretic, but did not know that she was not taking these tablets. He reasoned that if 80 mg furosemide was not clearing the fluid, he needed to give a much higher dose. If he had known that she had not been taking the tablets, he would not have done this. Mrs O could not tolerate the sudden introduction of a large dose of furosemide and sadly died. When her flat was cleared, her daughter found the unused tablets hidden in a cupboard.

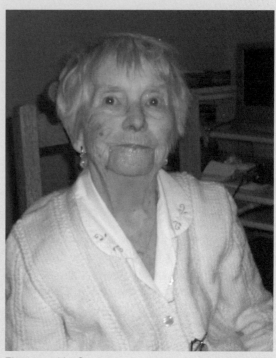

Figure 5.3 Mrs O.

coating (BNF, 2012). When a nurse is assessing a patient on admission it is important that they obtain a full medication history, including medicines that the patient has bought over the counter, or from the pharmacist, or health food shop.

Summary

Some patients are at more risk of adverse effects than others because they are more vulnerable. In this chapter we have examined many of the reasons why this is so, and what the alert nurse needs to consider in order to support patients to gain the maximum benefit from medications.

While the adjustment of treatment is generally a matter for prescribers, a nurse's knowledge and their professional contribution in supporting patients' medication management and optimization will help to ensure that those prescribers have the information they need to make optimal decisions for patients.

Further reading

Department of Health (2004), *Building a safer NHS for patients: Improving Medication Safety:* http://www.dh.gov.uk/prod_consum_dh/groups/dh_digitalassets/@dh/@en/documents/digitalasset/dh_4084961.pdf (accessed 16 December 2012).

Healy D (2008), *Psychiatric Drugs Explained*, 5th ed. Churchill Livingstone: Oxford.

References

Armour D, and Cairns C (2002), *Medicines in the Elderly*. London: Pharmaceutical Press.

Berlin CM (2009), *Pharmacokinetics in Children*. Available at: http:www.merck.com/mmpe/sec19/ch270/ch270b.html (accessed 16 December 2009).

BNF see Joint Formulary Committee.

Boyd CM, Darer J, Boult C, Fried LP, Boult L, and Wu AW (2005), Clinical practice guidelines and quality of care for older patients with multiple comorbid diseases; implications for pay for performance, *JAMA*, 294: 716–724.

Children Act 1989: c.41 (1989), London: The Stationery Office.

Conroy S, Choonara I, Impicciatore P, Mohn A, Arnell H, Anders R, et al (2000), Survey of unlicensed and off label drug use in paediatric wards in European countries, *BMJ*, 320; 79–82.

Department of Health (2001), *National Service Framework for Older People*. London: The Stationery Office.

Gidal B. (2006), Drug Absorption in the elderly: Biopharmaceutical considerations for the anti-epileptic drugs. *Epilepsy Research*, 68; 65–69.

Gurwitz J, and Avorn J (1991), The Ambiguous Relationship between Aging and Adverse Drug Reactions. *Annals of Internal Medicine*, 114; 956–966 Available at: http://www.annals.org/content/114/11/956.short (accessed: 4 May 2012).

Hafeez S, Sharma RA, Huddart RA, Dearnaley DP, and Horwich A. (2007). Challenges in treating patients with Down's syndrome and testicular cancer with chemotherapy and radiotherapy: The Royal Marsden experience. *Clinical Oncology*, 19; 135–142.

Hilmer SN (2008), The dilemma of polypharmacy. *Australian Prescriber*, 31; 2–3.

Hippisley-Cox J, Pringle M, and Ronan R (2004), Polypharmacy in the elderly: analysis of Q research data: http://www.qresearch.org/Public_Documents/DataValidation/Polypharmacy%20in%20the%20elderly.pdf?Source=httP%3A%2F%2Fwww%2Eqresearch%2Eorg%2FPublic%5FDocuments%2FForms%2FDispForm%2Easpx%3FID%3D18 (accessed 16 December 2012).

Joint Formulary Committee (2012), *British National Formulary* (64th ed). London: BMJ Group and Pharmaceutical Press.

Koh Y, Kutty FBM, and Li SC (2005), Drug-related problems in hospitalized patients on polypharmacy: the influence of age and gender, *Therapeutics and Cinical Risk Management*, 1; 39–48.

Lazarou J, Bruce H, Pomeranz MD, and Corey P (1998), Incidence of adverse drug reactions in hospitalized patients. A meta-analysis of prospective studies. *JAMA*, 279; 1200–1205.

Lindeman RD (1992), Changes in renal function with aging. Implications for treatment. *Drugs and Aging*, 2; 423–431.

Mangoni A, and Jackson S (2004), Age-related changes in pharmacokinetics and pharmacodynamics: basic principles and practical applications, *British Journal of Clinical Pharmacology*, 57; 6–14.

McGavock H (2010), *How Drugs Work. Basic Pharmacology for Health Professionals*. Oxford: Radcliffe Medical Press.

Neale G, Woloshynowych M, and Vincent C (2001), Exploring the causes of adverse events in NHS hospitals. *Journal of the Royal Society of Medicine*, 94; 322–330.

Nursing and Midwifery Council (2008), *The Code: Standards of Conduct, Performance and Ethics for Nurses and Midwives*. London: NMC.

Nursing and Midwifery Council (2010), *Standards for Medicines Management*. London: NMC.

Paediatric Formulary Committee (2012), *BNF for Children* (2012–2013). London: BMJ Group, Pharmaceutical Press, and RCPCH Publications.

Porth CM, Gaspard KJ, and Noble KA (2010), *Essentials of Pathophysiology: Concepts of Altered Health States*. Philadelphia: Lippincott, Williams and Wilkins.

Scott KM, Von Korff J, Alonso MC, Angermeyer E, Bromet J, Fayyad G, et al (2009), Mental –Physical co-morbidity and its relationship with disability: results from the World Mental Health Surveys. *Psychological Medicine*, 39; 33–43.

Smith D (2001), Health care management of adults with Down syndrome, *American Family Physician*, 64; 1031–1039.

St-Onge MP (2005), Relationship between body composition changes and changes in physical function and metabolic risk factors in aging. *Current Opinion in Clincal Nutrition and Metabolic Care*, 8; 523–528.

Tessier D, Dawson K, Tétrault JP, Bravo G, and Meneilly GS (1994), Glibenclamide vs gliclazide in type 2 diabetes of the elderly. *Diabetic Medicine*. 11; 974–980.

Thomson A (2004), Variability in drug dosage requirements. *Pharmaceutical Journal*, 272; 806–808.

Turnheim K (2003), When drug therapy gets old: pharmacokinetics and pharmacodynamics in the elderly. *Experimental Gerontology*, 38; 843–853.

Veehof LJ, Stewart RE, Meyboom-de JB, and Haaijer-Ruskamp FM (1999), Adverse drug reactions and polypharmacy in the elderly in general practice. *European Journal of Clinical Pharmacology*, 5; 533–536.

Vissink A, Karst F, Spijkervet l, and Amerongen N (1996), Aging and saliva: A review of the literature. *Special Care in Dentistry*, 16; 95–103.

Wallace SM, and Verbeeck RV (1987), Plasma protein binding of drugs in the elderly. *Clinical Pharmacokinetics*, 12; 41–72.

6 Information and Evidence: Sources and Evaluation

CHAPTER CONTENTS

- Information sources
- Assessing, critiquing, and critical appraisal
- *The British National Formulary* (BNF)

- Understanding evaluations
- Summary

LEARNING OUTCOMES

By the end of this chapter, you should understand

- The range of possible sources of information about medicines
- Their positive and negative characteristics
- Some trustworthy sources of evidence
- The role of medicines information departments
- Some basic principles of critical analysis of evidence
- How the *British National Formulary* (BNF) is structured
- How to read a BNF monograph
- A selection of terms used in the literature about medicines.

While nurses will not usually be selecting medicines, they still need information to make the best use of the medicines prescribed for their patients. Information of all kinds is much more readily available today than it was a generation ago when the authors were students, but much of it is of low quality and today's student must learn to test the quality of the evidence offered to see if it can be relied upon.

In all fields of healthcare it has become usual to insist that practice must be evidence based. This is very desirable, but it begs the question—what is evidence?

This chapter will examine some of the sources of evidence about medicines that are available and give some guidance on their reliability. Later, there will be an introduction to critical analysis of sources, and a description of some of the key terms used in evaluating clinical evidence about medicines.

Information sources

Sources of information may be conveniently divided into two main types—people and publications. It is natural that many healthcare professionals should rely upon their mentors and instructors to supplement the knowledge they gain in formal teaching. Indeed, for many years much of the practical information about medicines that junior doctors received came from participation in ward rounds under the tutelage of a consultant. In medical school they learned some general pharmacology, but the actions of many drugs were learned following graduation (Maxwell and Walley, 2009)

The same will be true for nurses, and it will continue to be true throughout their careers. New medicines will come into use, and nurses will have to learn about them. It is therefore important to realize that pharmacology will be a lifelong study and does not end with registration as a nurse. Moreover, for many nurses there will be a degree of specialization, but a basic competence is expected in all areas. For example, a nurse specializing in cardiac rehabilitation will probably need a level of knowledge about the medicines they use that is similar to that of a general practitioner, but they will know rather less about other medicines. However, they will still need to know something about other drugs that their patients may have for co-existing medical conditions.

Given the need to gain and maintain a competence in medicines, which sources can a student nurse rely upon? Fortunately there are many sources and some clear guidance to their relative reliability.

First, fact is to be preferred to opinion. Sometimes it is not easy to tell the two apart. For example, many guidelines are a mixture of the two. They use facts for those parts of the care pathway where there is strong evidence, but since they need to give a complete pathway they must fill the gaps with expert opinion. While the majority is not always right, experience tells us that a consensus amongst a group is more likely to be right than a single person's opinion, so if we lack facts, a consensus of experts is the next best option. (NICE, 2005, especially Table 7.1)

As in everyday life, we are more inclined to believe something is correct if we have a number of sources saying the same thing. We must be careful not to confuse this with many reports that ultimately come from one source. A press release may be reported in a number of newspapers, radio and television programmes, and be repeated many times, but there is actually only one source for that story.

Appraising the evidence for a medicine's effectiveness therefore involves at least two steps; we must collect evidence using some type of **structured search**, and we must evaluate its quality.

Where can good evidence be found?

This is such an important subject that the Department of Health has sponsored a number of bodies to create, record, and evaluate good quality clinical evidence. It is important to busy health professionals to have information that they can trust so that they do not have to perform the evidence gathering and evaluation themselves. A few examples of such bodies are listed here, with a description of the work they do.

The Centre for Reviews and Dissemination (CRD) is part of the National Institute for Health Research (NIHR) and is part of the University of York. CRD was established in 1994 and its job is to collect and review health-related evidence systematically. It has published a helpful—though detailed—free guide to performing such a review on its website: *Systematic Reviews: CRD's guidance for undertaking reviews in health care*, at: **http://www.york.ac.uk/inst/crd/ index_guidance.htm**.

Not all of its work is related to medicines. For example, in 2009 it published a study testing how increasing the price of cigarettes would reduce smoking (CRD, 2008).

Another important part of the National Institute for Health Research is the **Health Technology Assessment** programme (HTA) which is run by the NIHR Evaluation, Trials, and Studies Coordinating Centre (NETSCC) based at the University of Southampton. HTA produces research about the effectiveness of treatments and tests for the NHS. Having identified questions that need asking, it then commissions research to provide answers. It also examines the same question from different approaches. For example, in 2010 it published a report on *The safety and effectiveness of different methods of ear wax removal: a systematic review and economic evaluation*. This looked at the evidence for the best and safest method, but also the cheapest and most cost-effective. HTA's publications can be downloaded free from the internet at: **http://www.hta. nhs.uk/project/htapubs.asp**.

HTA does a substantial amount of work for the **National Institute for Health and Clinical Excellence** (NICE), which is perhaps the best known of the evidence sifting bodies. NICE's job is not to answer questions of purely academic interest, but to provide independent national guidance on promoting good health and preventing and treating ill health. It publishes a range of outputs. Some are clinical guidelines looking at the care of patients with a particular condition. Others are technology appraisals, which are examinations of the effectiveness and cost-effectiveness of treatments. If a NICE technology appraisal rules that a treatment should be made available, NHS organizations are obliged to offer it within three months. (Newdick, 2005)

When NICE publishes guidance it also releases the evidence upon which it was based, and grades the quality of that evidence. It publishes a very comprehensive manual on the way that it grades and uses evidence, which can be seen at: **http://www.nice.org. uk/aboutnice/howwework/developingniceclinical- guidelines/clinicalguidelinedevelopmentmethods/ GuidelinesManual2009.jsp**.

NICE's remit does not extend to Scotland, where similar work is undertaken by two bodies. The **Scottish Medicines Consortium** examines new treatments and advises NHS Boards in Scotland as to whether the NHS should adopt them. Their decisions can be found at: **http://www.scottishmedicines.org**.

The **Scottish Intercollegiate Guidelines Network** (SIGN) produces evidence-based clinical guidelines for use by the NHS in Scotland. The quality of its work is acknowledged to be good, so some English NHS organizations will use SIGN guidelines while they wait for a judgement from NICE. SIGN's website is at: **http:// www.sign.ac.uk**.

The multiplicity of sources of evidence has led the Department of Health to give NICE the task of setting up and running **NHS Evidence**. NHS Evidence is a single portal to around 150 sources of information so that all health and social care staff have free access to best-practice information that has been checked by experts. NHS Evidence is building specialist libraries in some areas, and accrediting some guidance producers so users know that their work can be trusted.

No survey of evidence sources would be complete without mention of the **Cochrane Collaboration**. The Cochrane Collaboration is an association of volunteers worldwide who work together to produce evidence-based guidelines. As an international body it avoids some of the pitfalls that other organizations face, because it can evaluate evidence that is not published in English. It takes its name from Professor Archie Cochrane, who was very influential in promoting the systematic and scientific analysis of medical trial work. Its website is at: **http://www. cochrane.org**.

UKMi

UKMi (note the lower case i) is the abbreviation for the United Kingdom Medicines Information service. Most hospital trusts have a medicines information department—around 250 across the UK—with ten regional centres and national centres for Northern Ireland and Wales. They answer enquiries from other healthcare professionals on all aspects of drug therapy, and in an average year they will collectively handle about half a million queries. The local centres support ward pharmacists and may have responsibility for compiling the local medicines formulary and providing expertize to Drug and Therapeutics Committees.

In addition to this local work, the regional centres often have a role in education and training, and some are Poisons Information Centres. Regional centres also specialize, and in this way they can support colleagues in other parts of the country. The current specialist centres are shown in Table 6.1.

Comprehensive contact details for all UKMi centres can be found at: **http://www.ukmi.nhs.uk/ukmi/ directory/default.asp** which also contains a large store of resources relating to medicines, including over two hundred answers to questions that have been asked before. These answers are reviewed at intervals to keep them current.

The **National Prescribing Centre (NPC)** is, as its name suggests, an organization devised to help prescribers, but its resources are freely available to anyone, and these include substantial information on evidence-based therapeutics and medicines management. There is an interactive learning site (NPCi) which can be accessed through the main NPC website at: **http://www.npc.co.uk**.

Table 6.1 Specialist medicines information centres.

Subject	Centre
Alternative medicines	Welsh Medicines Information Centre, Cardiff
Drugs in porphyria	Welsh Medicines Information Centre, Cardiff
Drugs in breast milk	West Midlands Medicines Information Service, Sutton Coldfield
	Trent Medicines Information Centre, Leicester
Drugs in children	Alder Hey Hospital (Royal Liverpool Children's Trust)
Drugs in dentistry	North West Medicines Information Centre, Liverpool
Drugs in oncology	The Royal Marsden Hospital
Drugs in ophthalmology	Moorfields Eye Hospital
Drugs in pregnancy	Wolfson Unit, Newcastle upon Tyne
Drugs in psychiatry	The Maudsley Hospital, London
Drugs in renal disease	South West Medicines Information and Training, Bristol
Toxicology and poisoning	Regional Medicines and Poisons Information Centre, Belfast

NPC also publishes the MeRec bulletins, which appear monthly and consider the evidence behind topics, some of which have been suggested by NICE. For example, the MeReC monthly bulletin for March 2012 includes an article entitled 'Accredited guidance on combined hormonal and emergency contraception'. In April 2012 NPC was merged within NICE as part of the Evidence and Practice Directorate under the new title NICE Medicines and Prescribing Centre. The NPC websites remain as legacy sites but will be transferred to the NICE site: **www.nice.nhs.uk** in due course.

One of the early sources of unbiased information about medicines was the **Drug and Therapeutics Bulletin (DTB)** which is now published by the BMJ Group. Access is by subscription, but NHS staff with Athens accounts can access it free of charge, and there is also a free downloadable monthly podcast. In common with the other resources listed, it does not accept advertising or sponsorship and has consequently been run on a very low budget.

A group of doctors and medical scientists based in Oxford started a journal devoted to evidence-based medicine in 1994. The paper journal was called **Bandolier** and its approach and style made it a little easier to read than DTB. The paper version is no longer produced, but there is now an electronic journal accessible at: **http://www.medicine.ox.ac.uk/bandolier**.

They also produce some books that explore topics in more depth. For example, Bandolier has published *Bandolier's Little Book of Pain* (2003) which summarizes a large amount of evidence about various types of pain and its treatment.

This list is not exhaustive, and there are many other excellent resources that can be trusted. Experienced colleagues working in different fields of practice will have their own favourites, and it is always worth asking them for suggestions. However, you must make up your own mind about their impartiality and accuracy, and later in this chapter we will consider how to do that.

Exercise 6.1

This would be a good point to pause to consider what factors you would need to think about when deciding whether to trust a resource. Make a list now, and check it against our suggestions later.

Using the internet

As with other subjects, there are many sources of information about medicines on the internet, and their quality ranges from very helpful and reliable, to completely misleading rubbish. In general, it is easier to evaluate websites based in and written for the United Kingdom, but there are some useful sources in English published in other countries. For example, in North America OTIS (the Organization of Teratology Information Specialists) available at: http://www.otispregnancy.org produces factsheets on the effects of some medicines on the fetus which supplement UK information sources. However, when a foreign source is used, you must remember that medicines' licences may be different abroad, so statements about doses, indications (reasons for use), and legal categories may not correspond to UK practice.

Similarly, a large number of patient and self-help groups publish information about medicines, some of which is very good. Diabetes UK at: http://www.diabetes.org.uk has a lot of useful information, including resources for you to give patients in languages other than English. One much-used resource is their Ramadan calendar, which gives the times of prayer during Ramadan alongside advice on managing diabetes during the daytime fast. Parkinson's UK has a lot of advice for patients with Parkinson's disease and those who provide care for them at: http://www.parkinsons.org.uk.

There are many other websites that are not evidence-based, some of which are frankly misleading. One pointer to the quality of the information offered is the name and qualifications of the people behind them. This is not always clear, but for Diabetes UK and Parkinson's UK the websites list the current trustees or advisers, amongst whom there are well-qualified healthcare professionals. It is unlikely that a senior doctor, nurse, or pharmacist with a reputation to lose would allow their name to be associated with a poor quality website.

The same is true of printed information. A reputable publisher, an author who is well-known and professionally qualified in a relevant area of practice and, ideally, a journal that subscribes to a code of practice, are all indicators that the text can be relied upon. The best type of journal is one in which the articles are **peer-reviewed**. This means that the author's essay will have been read by one or more experts who do not know who has written the article, so that they cannot be impressed by someone's reputation. If they think the article is of adequate quality, it will be published; if not, it is returned to the author with suggestions for improvement.

The editors of nearly a thousand medical and nursing journals are members of **WAME** (pronounced whammy), the World Association of Medical Editors. This exists to improve quality and ethical standards in medical publishing. Its members are listed at: http://www.wame.org.

If you use a journal on that list, you can be sure that it generally meets high standards—though it is still possible that an author may have misled them. The International Committee of Medical Journal Editors (ICMJE) has a similar aim and publishes standards for manuscript submission at: http://www.icmje.org.

To take just a couple of standards, ICMJE requires authors to disclose who paid for their research work, so readers know if the paper is likely to be biased, and the authors must include a statement that humans or animals have not been maltreated in their research or, if this was unavoidable, that a responsible body agreed that this was the case. As a general rule, you can assume that journals whose editors belong to one or other of these bodies are taking care not to publish unreliable material.

Assessing, critiquing, and critical appraisal

There are formal tools available in the form of checklists and scoring charts that help professionals to assess the quality of the sources they use. For example, Solutions for Public Health publishes its Critical Appraisal Skills Programme (CASP) which provides checklists for appraising different types of clinical paper. All these tools are available at: http://www.sph.nhs.uk/what-we-do/public-health-workforce/resources/critical-appraisals-skills-programme.

The first steps in appraisal are to ask ourselves three questions that tell us whether it is worth looking at the paper in more detail:

1 **Was the study valid?** If there are defects in the design of the study, the conclusions may be un-reliable. As a rule we should prefer well-designed studies to poorly-designed ones, but sometimes there is no alternative and this will be the best evidence available. One such example is that of rare cancers. Since the numbers of patients may be very small, the patients may have to be treated by different doctors in a number of hospitals, perhaps in many countries in order to put together a group large enough to draw conclusions from. Each patient can only be treated once, so we cannot conduct some types of trial that allow the use of more than one treatment in the same patient, and it would not be ethical to give some of the patients a placebo just to allow a comparison. For all these reasons, the trial's validity may be questionable, but it can hardly be otherwise, and we would use the results whilst acknowledging that they may have defects.

2 **What results did it produce?** Surprisingly, some papers produce unclear or contradictory results. This must not be confused with negative results. A finding that a treatment did not work is still very useful and journal editors are encouraged to pub-lish these so that negative results become known. Even in some well-known, large clinical trials there is argument about what results were found. For example, the West of Scotland Coronary Prevention Study examined whether lipid-lowering drugs could help reduce the incidence of coronary heart disease in a range of patient groups (Shepherd, 1995). For some time after publication, there was argument as to whether all the lipid lowering drugs were useful, or just particular examples; whether all that mat-tered was that cholesterol was lowered somehow, regardless of how it was done; whether the results applied only to white men, or to other ethnic and gender groups.

3 **Were the results relevant to the patients I am concerned with?** If your practice is in Liverpool a project on the treatment of indigenous African tribespeople may not be the best evidence you could have, since you will not have many of them amongst your patients. While that is an extreme case, this is a key question that is sometimes ignored. If we are comparing methods of treating patients immediately after a heart attack, and we find that a team in another area is having better results than we are, does that mean that their treat-ment is better, or could it be that because their area is urban and ours is rural, patients in the urban area arrive at the hospital by ambulance much earlier?

A subtler example is one where a condition is diag-nosed differently in two places. If we have a paper on the treatment of high blood pressure, it is important to check whether the authors' cut-off point for counting the pres-sure as high is one that we would accept. A number of papers that rank painkilling drugs use results obtained in patients after surgery. This is logical because it is rea-sonable to suppose that patients who have had the same operation ought to feel similar amounts of pain, which is otherwise difficult to check. The patients will only have a few days of treatment so the trial can be quite quick to conduct. However, if your patients have chronic pain it is not clear that these rankings are relevant, because you have to manage a different type of pain.

A more detailed account of critical appraisal is beyond the scope of this book, but there is an excellent resource for nursing students on a website maintained by Richard Ingram at: **http://www.richard-ingram.co.uk**.

The British National Formulary (BNF)

The *BNF* was originally a recipe book for doctors and pharmacists to make some standard medicines, but it has evolved over the last thirty years to become a much more comprehensive and useful resource, available both in hard copy and on the internet at: **http://www.bnf.org**.

There is also an application for smartphones. The hard copy *BNF* is issued twice a year. The online edition mirrors the paper version, but an update section allows more frequent updating. There is also a facility to allow users to request emails when updates are released.

The *BNF* consists of some preliminary material, fifteen chapters classifying drugs by the body systems they work upon, nine appendices, and some miscellaneous topics. It is published twice a year, and helpfully each edition contains a summary near the front that describes what has changed since the last edition. This is followed by some advice for prescribers and some guidance on the management of poisoning.

The fifteen sections are arranged as follows:

1 Gastro-intestinal system

2 Cardiovascular system

3 Respiratory system

4 Central nervous system

5 Infections

6 Endocrine system

7 Obstetrics, gynaecology, and urinary-tract disorders

8 Malignant disease and immunosuppression

9 Nutrition and blood

10 Musculoskeletal and joint diseases

11 Eye

12 Ear, nose, and oropharynx

13 Skin

14 Immunological products and vaccines

15 Anaesthesia.

Each of these is then sub-divided. Chapter 1 on gastro-intestinal medicine is broken down into nine sub-sections:

1.1 Dyspepsia and gastro-oesophageal reflux disease

1.2 Antispasmodics and other drugs altering gut motility

1.3 Antisecretory drugs and mucosal protectants

1.4 Acute diarrhoea

1.5 Chronic bowel disorders

1.6 Laxatives

1.7 Local preparations for anal and rectal disorders

1.8 Stoma care

1.9 Drugs affecting intestinal secretions.

There is a further sub-division of each of these sections. Section 1.6 on laxatives is divided thus:

1.6.1 Bulk-forming laxatives

1.6.2 Stimulant laxatives

1.6.3 Faecal softeners

1.6.4 Osmotic laxatives

1.6.5 Bowel cleansing preparations

1.6.6 Peripheral opioid-receptor antagonists.

Beneath this level we come to the individual drugs. If we examine 1.6.2 on stimulant laxatives we come to:

Bisacodyl

Dantron

Docusate sodium

Glycerol

Senna

Sodium picosulfate

Other stimulant laxatives.

Drug monographs

All the monographs have a standard layout to make it easier to find the information that you want quickly.

Indications medical conditions for which the drug is used	
Cautions	reasons why the medicine may need to be used with extra care
Contra-indications	reasons why a medicine should either not be used or used only under the supervision of a specialist
Pregnancy	whether and when a drug can be used in pregnant women
Breast-feeding	whether a drug can be given to nursing mothers
Side-effects	the adverse effects that are known to occur with the medicine, listed in descending order of likelihood. This does not mean that rarer effects are unimportant!

This structure is shown by the monograph for senna.

> SENNA
>
> | | |
> |---|---|
> | Indications | constipation |
> | Cautions | see notes above |
> | Contra-indications | see notes above |
> | Pregnancy | see pregnancy |
> | Breast-feeding | not known to be harmful |
> | Side-effects | see notes above |
> | Dose | see under preparations |
> | Note | Acts in 8–12 hours. |

In order to reduce duplication, where information is shared by all the members of a group of drugs it may be given in the introduction to that section rather than each drug in turn. This explains the references to 'notes above' and 'see pregnancy'. At the end of the monograph there will be details of the brands or preparations available. For senna these include:

> **Senna (Non-proprietary)**
>
> *Tablets*, total sennosides (calculated as sennoside B) 7.5 mg. Net price 60 = £2.13
>   **Dose**
>   2–4 tablets, usually at night; initial dose should be low then gradually increased; child (but see section 1.6) 6–12 years, half adult dose in the morning (on doctor's advice only)
>   **Note**
>   Lower dose on packs on sale to the public
>   Brands include *Senokot*® NHS

The last symbol indicates that the Senokot brand cannot be prescribed in the community.

The nine appendices in the *BNF* give information about topics that cross the body systems approach of the main chapters. These appendices have undergone a radical change from *BNF 59* (March 2010). The numbering is unaltered but the text that used to be in appendices 2–5 has been transferred to the relevant drug entries, so if you want to know about the use of senna in pregnancy, you now look in the entry for senna, rather than in the appendix about pregnancy.

Appendix 1 Interactions

Appendix 2 Liver disease

Appendix 3 Renal impairment

Appendix 4 Pregnancy

Appendix 5 Breast-feeding

Appendix 6 Intravenous additives

Appendix 7 Borderline substances

Appendix 8 Wound management products and elasticated garments

Appendix 9 Cautionary and advisory labels for dispensed medicines.

The *BNF for Children* (BNFC) is organized in the same way, with the same chapter numbers, but there are only four appendices:

Appendix 1 Interactions

Appendix 2 Borderline substances

Appendix 3 Cautionary and advisory labels for dispensed medicines

Appendix 4 Intravenous infusions for neonatal intensive care.

Understanding evaluations

This textbook is not primarily designed to teach critical appraisal, but there are some terms used in papers that need to be understood.

A common way of expressing the effectiveness of a medicine in a clinical trial is to give the **number needed to treat (NNT)**. If you have two matching groups of patients and give one drug A while the other is given a dummy tablet, then the NNT is the number of patients that you need in each group in order to prevent one additional bad outcome. For example, if drug A is meant to prevent heart attacks, and you have 3 patients out of 100 in that group who suffer an attack in two years, while 4 out of 100 suffer a heart a attack when given the placebo (dummy tablet), then the NNT is 100—the number of patients who had to receive drug A in order to prevent one extra heart attack.

An important point to note is that NNTs are linked to treatment times. In our example, the NNT was 100 over

2 years. If you give the drug for less than two years, you would expect the results not to be as good, and the NNT would rise—you would need more patients to compensate for the shorter time. To allow differing trials to be compared, some writers use annualized NNTs, which are simply the NNT multiplied by the length of the trial in years—in the case of our example, $100 \times 2 = 200$.

The best possible NNT would be 1. For that to happen, all the patients in the control group would have to fail to improve, while all the patients in treatment group became better. The higher the NNT, the less effective the drug is, because you have to treat more people to achieve one success.

A related descriptor is the **number needed to harm (NNH)**, which looks at the number of patients that have to be treated with the new drug before one extra patient suffers a particular side effect. In this case, a large number is obviously to be preferred, because it is better if you can treat a hundred patients before one suffers an adverse event than if you can only treat ten.

These two factors can be compared. For instance, if we have a new drug to treat migraine that can be shown to cause fits in some patients, we need to know whether the added benefit (less migraine) is worth the added risk (more fits). If the NNT is 12, but the NNH is 8, then more patients will have an adverse effect than will have a beneficial one, so we would probably not use that drug. However, it is not quite as simple as that. If the benefit is very great, and the risk is unimportant, it may still be worth giving that medicine. Many anticancer drugs cause nausea and vomiting, and the success rate with some of them is not very high, so the NNH may be a low number when the NNT is much higher, but because nausea is much less important to most patients than surviving their cancer, the treatment may still be offered.

The results of clinical trials may also be expressed as **risk reductions**. Drug companies often want to promote their drugs using **relative risk reductions (RRR)**. These make the effect of the drug look much more impressive, but may be misleading if the event you are trying to avoid is very rare. The **absolute risk reduction (ARR)** more clearly indicates the real change that has taken place. An example may help to explain this.

Let us consider a trial in which the investigators want to know whether giving a lipid lowering drug to patients who have never had a heart attack will reduce their risk of suffering one later. They divide their patients into two groups. The experimental group receives the drug, and the control group receives a dummy tablet. In each case the study lasts for three years. At the end of that time, 1.7% of the patients receiving the drug have had a heart attack, against 2.7% in the control group. The relative risk reduction is therefore $(2.7 - 1.7) / 2.7 = 37\%$, which looks very impressive. However, the absolute risk reduction is only $2.7 - 1.7 = 1\%$, because heart attacks in these patients were quite rare.

This is clearly shown when the NNT is calculated. Since the absolute risk reduction is 1%, the investigators had to treat 100 patients to reduce the number of heart attacks by 1, so the NNT over three years is 100. Seen from this perspective, treating 100 patients for 3 years to prevent 1 heart attack may not be a good use of NHS resources. A patient who was offered this drug might feel that taking a tablet for the rest of his life in order to ward off an unlikely event was not something that he wanted to do.

An alternative measure that is sometimes used, and that some authors think is better understood by some patients, is the **odds ratio**. This compares the chance that something will happen in the treated patients with the chance that it will happen in the patients given the control treatment. In our example, this would be $1.7 / 2.7 = 0.63$. However, this again ignores the scale of the risk, because it is a relative measure, not an absolute one. It does not tell us what risk the patient is actually running, just that it is around two-thirds as large when they take this drug as it would have been without it.

Summary

This chapter has given an introduction to sources of evidence about medicines that can be relied upon, and suggested how others can be evaluated. The *British National Formulary* is a readily available standard source and its structure has been described to assist in its use. Finally, a few basic terms used in assessing drug treatments have been described.

References

BNF see Joint Formulary Committee.

Centre for Reviews and Dissemination (CRD) (2008), *Population tobacco control interventions and their effects on social inequalities in smoking*. CRD Report 39. York: University of York. Also available at: http://www.york.ac.uk/inst/crd/CRD_Reports/crdreport39.pdf (accessed 1 June 2012).

Joint Formulary Committee (2012). *British National Formulary* (64th ed). London: BMJ Group and Pharmaceutical Press.

Maxwell S and Walley T (2009), Teaching safe and effective prescribing in UK medical schools: a core curriculum for tomorrow's doctors, *Br J Clin Pharmacol*, 55; 496–503.

National Institute for Health and Clinical Excellence (NICE) (2005), *Guideline Development Methods: 7 Reviewing and grading the evidence*, available at: http://www.nice.org.uk/niceMedia/pdf/GDM_Chapter7_0305.pdf (accessed 1 June 2012).

Newdick C (2005), Who should we treat? (2nd ed), Oxford University Press: Oxford, pp 206–207.

Shepherd J et al for the West of Scotland Coronary Prevention Study Group (1995), Prevention of coronary heart disease with pravastatin in men with hypercholesterolaemia, *New England Journal of Medicine* 333; pp 1301–1307.

Paediatric Formulary Committee (2012), *BNF for Children* (2012–2013). London: BMJ Group, Pharmaceutical Press, and RCPCH Publications.

7 Medicines Management: Systems and Procedures

CHAPTER CONTENTS

- Why do we need systems and procedures?
- Medicines management: definitions
- Components of medicines management
- Standards for medicines management
- Responsibility
- Accountability
- Stock management
- One stop dispensing
- Reducing risk by proper organization of stock cupboards and drug trolleys
- Medicines administration records and record keeping
- What is medicines reconciliation?
- Taking a medicines history on admission: the acquisition of necessary practical skills
- Quiz
- National standards for medicines management
- The role of the Care Quality Commission
- Summary

LEARNING OUTCOMES

By the end of this chapter you should be able to:

- Understand the responsibilities and accountability of the student and trained nurse with regards to medicines management
- Understand the reasons for policy to support medicines management
- Interpret the role of the nurse in relation to policies and standards for medicines management
- Understand the role of the nurse in relation to key standards and drivers for the safer administration and management of medicines.

The aims of this chapter are to support you to interpret the responsibility that you already carry as a student and will carry as a registrant when giving medicines to patients and to help you to understand what is meant by accountability and how this relates to your role now and in the future in the management of medicines.

Medicines management occurs wherever there is a patient and is carried out in a variety of settings which include:

- acute hospitals
- community hospitals
- care homes, both residential care homes and nursing homes

- the patient's own home
- schools
- community clinics.

Exercise 7.1

> Can you think of any other settings that are not listed here?

Why do we need systems and procedures?

The National Patient Safety Agency (NPSA, 2004) has produced guidance for organizations on supporting patient safety. They suggested the implementation of seven steps as follows:

1 Build a safety culture.

2 Lead and support your staff.

3 Integrate your risk management activity.

4 Promote reporting.

5 Involve and communicate with patients and the public.

6 Learn and share safety lessons.

7 Implement solutions to prevent harm.

When interpreted in relation to medicines management and nursing care this means that the employing organization has a duty of care to its employees and patients to ensure that medicines are dispensed, supplied, and administered safely and that procedures are in place to support this. Managers need to be made aware of anything that might prevent this, and must ensure that checks are in place to prevent harm from occurring. The clear and prompt reporting of concerns, risk, and errors to management is pivotal to patient safety and medicines management in nursing and, from an organizational point of view, patient consultation and involvement is vital. Lessons must be shared in a 'low blame culture' and changes made to support the reduction of risk and potential harm. For more on communication and on risk reduction please see Chapters 1 and 10.

Medicines are important for improving patients' conditions. They can help by eradicating viral and bacterial infection, supporting the management of long-term conditions, eliminating acute and chronic pain, curing life threatening illnesses such as some cancers and enhancing quality of life. However, they can also cause great harm.

The giving of medicines to patients or advising patients on how, when, where, and how long to take their medicines is arguably one of the most important roles of the nurse. Published research estimates that approximately 247 000 (6.5%) hospital admissions in England each year are due to harm from medicines, of which 9% were preventable and 63% were possibly preventable (NPSA, 2009).

Exercise 7.2

> When in practice ask your mentor to show you the medicines policy. Discuss this with your mentor in relation to the role of the nurse.
>
> What does the medicines policy say about the role of the trained nurse?
>
> What does it say about the role of the student nurse?

Medicines management: definitions

The management of medicines incorporates many different facets. Broadly, the term means understanding how to use medicines safely, economically, ethically, within the law, within local and national policies, standards, and guidelines, and to best effect. There is no point and it would not be safe to practise one of the above without the others. The National Prescribing Centre defines medicines management as: 'a system of processes and behaviours that determines how medicines are used by patients and by the NHS' (NPC, 2002).

Increasingly the term 'medicines optimization' is being used. This reminds us that the activity is intended to obtain maximum benefit for the patient, and is therefore patient-centred, rather than concentrating on the medicines.

Historically, medicines management has been expressed in terms of five rights—giving the right medicine to the right patient at the right time by the right route and in the right dose. Recently this has been expanded and some others now list nine rights (Elliott and Liu, 2010) as described in Table 7.1

Components of medicines management

Medicines management is a multifaceted or umbrella concept, with variations of meaning according to the setting and, perhaps, the profession. Its purpose is to safeguard the patient and ensure the maximum benefit from their medication. As such it embraces a range of

Table 7.1 The nine 'rights' of medicine administration.

Right patient	The medicine must be given to the person for whom it is prescribed
Right drug	The patient must be given the correct medicine
Right route	The person administering the medicine must use the prescribed route (for example, subcutaneous injection rather than intramuscular)
Right time	The dose must be given at the right time, not only by the clock but also with reference to meals or procedures
Right dose	The right amount of the medicine must be given
Right documentation	The action of giving medication must be properly evidenced on the patient's medicines administration record, but may also have to be recorded elsewhere, such as a Controlled Drugs register
Right action	The nurse should check that the reason for giving the medicine is correct. For example, if a patient has diarrhoea but has been prescribed a laxative this should be checked
Right form	The medicine must be in the appropriate form for the route. An oral syrup cannot be injected, for example
Right response	The nurse should monitor the patient for signs of the expected response to the medication and report unexpected responses.

actions, not all of which are engaged in on every patient contact. Some of these actions are concerned with the way that systems support the supply of medicines. The following list shows the complexity of the actions needed to ensure good medicines management. Although some have been assigned to particular settings for convenience, most of these are continuing activities and have to be reviewed throughout the patient journey.

During the initial consultation:

- Deciding whether a medicine is needed.
- Selecting appropriate treatment.
- Involving patients in the choice of treatment, respecting their views and priorities and enabling them to take a more active role in self-management.
- Providing patient-centred information.
- Using non-pharmacological options where possible, including health promotion advice.

At later consultations:

- Monitoring for benefits and safety.
- Reviewing effectiveness of treatment.
- Deciding when to stop treatment.
- Identifying under-treatment as well as over-treatment.

Throughout the healthcare community:

- Reducing medicines wastage.
- Improving repeat prescribing systems.
- Developing patient-friendly ordering and collection systems.
- Promoting better communication between prescribers, patients, carers, and other health professionals.
- Making the best use of resources—evidence-based formularies and guidelines; generic prescribing; synchronization of quantities; medicines no longer needed; optimization of doses.
- Identifying further areas of investment in treatments to produce improved health outcomes, for example prescribing aspirin or statins in patients at risk of coronary heart disease.
- Using professionals appropriately.

Managing demand (DH 2004a).

There are obvious linkages between some of these. Choosing the appropriate medicine for the patient will be informed by evidence-based formularies and guidelines, and those in turn respond to the need to invest for better outcomes. One aspect of managing demand is to ensure that the patient sees the most appropriate professional and this is where you as a nurse will be involved.

Exercise 7.3

Consider which of these relate to the role of the nurse and which are managed either individually or jointly with other members of the multi-disciplinary team (MDT).

Reflection point

- From your observations, how are members of the MDT involved in the administration of medicines?
- Who else might be part of the MDT?
- How do members of the MDT communicate with each other?

Reflect on a situation you might have observed in practice relating to medicines management and the MDT. What went well? What could have been improved? How could you use this learning to influence your future practice?

Standards for medicines management

The NMC (2010) has provided a set of minimum practice standards to which all registered nurses who are giving medicines must work. These are underpinned by the NMC (2008) *Code of Conduct, Performance and Ethics*. The standards also apply to students who have been delegated by a registered professional to supply or administer a medicinal product. Within these standards it is implicit that patient safety is of the highest importance.

Who can administer medicines?

Nurses do not administer medicines in isolation and the registered nurse is part of a multidisciplinary team (MDT), members of which include:

- The doctor
- The pharmacist
- Registered pharmacy technicians
- Allied registered health professionals such as the physiotherapist, podiatrist, radiographer, and paramedic
- Assistant practitioners.

The Department of Health (2006) *Medicine Matters: A guide to mechanisms for prescribing, supply and administration of medicines*, section 11, states that:

Any suitably trained member of staff in health or social care can administer medicines that have been prescribed, by an authorized prescriber, for an individual patient. The medicines can then only be given to that named patient. This principle applies to registered and non-registered staff at all levels. However, non-registered staff cannot administer medicines using a patient group directive, and cannot train to prescribe medicines.

The NMC (2008) adds that the administration of medicines 'requires thought and professional judgement' (NMC, 2008, p 1.) Therefore registered nurses carry a responsibility for their actions and decisions and for those to whom they delegate.

Differences between supply and administration

The terms **supply** and **administration** are often misunderstood and interpreted to mean the same thing; however, they are different when applied in relation to the management of medicines.

Supply relates to the giving of medication to the patient or to the carer for them to take away and to administer over a period of time that is specified on the prescription.

Administration relates to the giving of the medicines to the patient, either for them to take themselves, immediately, or assisting them to take those medicines.

Similarly we need to distinguish between dispensing and prescribing.

Prescribing involves the selection of the right medicine by a qualified prescriber for the individual patient and the ordering of it through an appropriate process, usually involving a particular form such as an FP10 in the community or a prescription chart. There is no national prescription chart yet in England but there are a number of national charts in use in Wales, which can be seen at: **http://www.wales.nhs.uk/sites3/page.cfm?orgid=371andpid=47669**.

Dispensing is the provision of the medicine to the patient. In the case of a pharmacist this means giving the patient a medicine to take home for use, whereas to a nurse it will mean giving the medicine to the patient to take. To avoid confusion, we will use the word 'administration' for the act of giving medicine to a patient for immediate use, and reserve 'dispensing' for the process of preparing medicines for the patient to take away, whether this is done by a pharmacist or a nurse. This usage is supported by the NMC in *Standards for medicine management (2010)*, section 2, which describes the circumstances in which a registered nurse can dispense medicines.

In all cases the person who is prescribing, supplying, or administering the drug must be competent to do so.

Responsibility

If you have responsibility it means that you are:

- Responsible for something or to someone and that you have been given a 'job' or 'duty' for which you are answerable (accountable), (NMC, 2008).

Within the definition there is an assumption that if you don't know what to do or how to do it you would say so. Registrants are responsible for their decisions and actions; this means that they are responsible for:

- Assessing what is in the best interests of patients,
- Taking/giving responsibility,
- Maintaining their knowledge base.

Accountability

The registrant is fully accountable for both the things that they do (their actions) and for the things that they do not do either deliberately or as a result of omissions. In the case of a student nurse, the mentor is responsible for ensuring that they are competent to perform the tasks that have been delegated to them. The registrant has an obligation to give an account of what has been done, and as such they must be able to defend their course of action to a higher authority (for example to their employer, the law, the patient, their professional body).

Ethical implications

The registered nurse will owe a duty of care to their patients and be accountable for everything that they do or don't do. In the words of the NMC (2008, p.2), nurses are accountable for their 'actions and omissions' to ensure that they:

- Practise in the best interests of their patients,
- Do no harm either deliberately or through negligence to their patients.

This means that all nurses, whether in training or when they are registered, must work with an awareness of the latest and best evidence-based practice and that they must work within local policies and guidelines. If they believe that these are incompatible—that is, local policies do not follow best practice—it is their responsibility to say so to their mentor or to their line manager.

When supplying, or administering medicines, nurses must only work within their field of competence and their scope of practice. Registered nurses are responsible for ensuring that those to whom they delegate the task of giving medicines to patients are competent, and they must ensure clear, accurate, and timely record keeping and communication. Decisions regarding the patient's medicine must ideally be made in partnership with the patient and/or their carer(s).

Legal implications

A mechanism to supply or administer a medicine is a framework within which the practitioner who is giving the medicine to the patient must work legally. The nurse must be aware of the different mechanisms that are in place for the supply and administration of medicines, for example by prescription only, by patient specific direction (PSD), by patient group direction (PGD), by pharmacy, and by general sales list. See Chapter 1 to revise this if necessary.

Remember that you cannot give a prescription only medicine or a pharmacy only medicine to a patient without authority to do so. That authority may be personal (a prescription or a patient specific direction) or an authority to give to a person falling within a group (patient group direction). Although it would be legal to give a general sales list medicine, employers usually have instructions in place to prevent this in order to ensure that the patient's medicines record is complete. If you become aware that a patient is receiving medicine, or is giving themselves medicine, that has not been prescribed within your hospital or other workplace, you must report the matter to your manager or supervisor.

Clinical governance

Registered nurses are required to work within the clinical governance framework of their employing organization. A registered nurse who is giving medicine to a patient will be responsible for their safety. The clinical governance framework is in place to protect the patient by ensuring that they are working within both local and national policy and to best evidence base with up-to-date, effective, and cost effective practice. A registered nurse is accountable to their employer, the Nursing and Midwifery Council, the public, and to the law. This means that they could be asked to give a rational explanation (be called to account) for their decisions and for their actions or inactions that could occur either deliberately or as a result of negligence. This will be considered further in Chapter 10.

When medicines are not given as planned, the nurse should make a report through the system specified by their employer. Occasionally the number of such reports in a hospital or Trust is commented upon in the press as evidence of poor practice. In fact, high reporting may demonstrate that practice is generally very good. One purpose of the reporting is to learn from our mistakes and high reporting levels support that. There may be good reasons for deviations from expectations. For example, a patient may not be on the ward at the time of a medicine round because they have been taken for an x-ray or other test; an experienced (registered) nurse may feel that a sleeping patient does not need to be woken to be given a sedative; or, perhaps, a competent patient does not want their medicine, which should be respected and recorded.

We all make mistakes. If we came to the end of our careers believing that we had not made any mistakes, that would probably tell us more about our poor reflective practice than our competence. The NHS cannot have a 'no blame' culture, as is sometimes talked about, because we must face the fact that a very small number of colleagues deserve blame. We should speak instead of 'fair blame' in which the aim is to learn from mishaps and to improve our practice. The culture within the NHS is to share that learning and to learn from others' mistakes as well as our own, so that we do not have to make mistakes before we question our own practice.

Reflection point

Think of a practical example where a mistake has been made regarding the supply or administration of medicine. Describe what happened, using the questions to guide you.

Who was involved?

How was it discovered?

Who reported it?

How was it investigated?

Which professionals were involved in the investigation or inquiry?

What were the learning points?

Was a training plan put in place as a result of the learning points?

Who was involved in the training?

How, if at all, was practice improved or changed as a result of these learning points?

It is not appropriate to give real examples from practice (practice areas might be identified breaking patient anonymity and confidentiality) (NMC 2008). The point is that mistakes often happen and that there is usually more than one person involved. It is important that we act in an open and honest way to share these errors and that we are supported by the workplace culture to learn from these mistakes and to improve practice to stop them from happening again.

Take time to think of your own examples and discuss these with your mentor or other colleagues.

Stock management

The starting point must be that there should be nothing on the ward, or in the patient's home, that will not be used. This enhances safety because a patient cannot take or be given the wrong medicine if it is not there to give. It is also desirable for the NHS, because medicines that will not be used represent waste, and the cost of wasted medicines is considerable (see Exercise 7.4). As a preliminary benchmark, the national cost of prescribing in primary care is currently about £8 billion per year (National Audit Office, 2007; Trueman et al, 2010) with drug wastage in the NHS in England being estimated at around £300 million per year (Trueman et al, 2010). Resources are finite and those that are wasted on unused medicines could have been better used elsewhere. Everyone has a responsibility to consider sustainability and to reduce wastage in everyday practice.

Depending upon the setting, you may have medicines labelled for the individual patient, or you may have a stock of medicines to be used as a need arises. For example, a minor injury unit will have small stocks of painkillers for those who attend. On most wards today, medicines are labelled for the individual patient. There are obvious advantages in having patient-labelled supplies. The appropriateness of the medicine for the patient has already been checked by the prescriber and by the pharmacist, which reduces the risk that a patient will be given something that they should not have. Provided there are local protocols to support this, these medicines may sometimes be given to patients on discharge, which means a new supply will not be needed. This again reduces waste and delay to the patient on discharge, and safeguards them against being given the wrong medicine at that stage by providing continuity of supply. Of course it is important that whoever is prescribing for the patient at discharge checks whether the medicines are still needed.

However, in some areas of practice this will not be easy to achieve. Areas of first contact with patients—accident and emergency departments, sexual health clinics, out of hours services, and others—may need to keep supplies for immediate supply or administration under a patient group direction or a patient specific direction (for revision of these terms please see Chapter 1).

You may hear colleagues talking about PODs, which is a common abbreviation for 'patient's own drugs'.

Exercise 7.4

What does sustainability in the workplace mean to you particularly in relation to medicines administration and management? How can nurses protect resources and reduce waste?

Points you might wish to consider:

- How often are patients' medicines reviewed?
- Are the quantities stocked sensible—sufficient to provide for the patient until the next review, but not so high that a lot will be wasted if the medication is changed? (Remember that a change of dose will

usually require the medicine to be returned to the pharmacy and a new supply with the correct instructions must be obtained.)

- What happens to medicines that are no longer needed by the patient?
- Who is responsible for the review of patients' medicines?
- How are patients' medicines packaged?
- What happens to discarded packaging?

The full term is preferable in case it is mistaken for a pod, meaning a small bedside container that some hospitals use to hold patients' possessions. The use of patients' own medicines is encouraged in hospitals. This reduces waste, should promote continuity, and improves adherence because the patient is already familiar with the medicines and their appearance. However, there should be procedures in place to assess the suitability of the PODs before they are used. These will differ between Trusts and you will need to familiarize yourself with the policy in your workplace. Do not assume that it is the same in all places, even within the same hospital group. Typically, the ward pharmacist will decide whether medicines may be used, having considered their condition, whether their identity is certain, how they have been stored, and whether the need for them to be continued has been established. For an explanation of the term adherence please see Chapter 9.

In hospitals, ward pharmacists and technicians play a vital role in the management of ward stock. Good stock management ensures that necessary medicines—but only the necessary ones—are in place for patients when they are needed. The importance of this is obvious when patients have labelled supplies, but it is also true for stock cupboards. An out-of-hours service that has no painkillers or antibiotics cannot offer a good service to the public.

Stock cupboards will usually have a list of items that are agreed as being likely to be needed in that setting, often with recommended quantities that have been agreed with the supplying pharmacy. Restocking systems vary, but nurses should take time to familiarize themselves with the system used in their workplace. For example, do you have to log stock items used as they are taken, or does someone count the stock at the end of each shift or day and place a top-up order?

One stop dispensing

Increasingly hospitals are switching to a new system described as 'one stop dispensing' where this is appropriate. This is designed to improve medicines management and reduce waste. Note that the main driver is to improve the management of medicines; its capacity to save money is a secondary benefit.

The logic behind one stop dispensing can be easily seen if we consider the traditional method of providing medicines. In the past, when a patient was admitted they were asked to surrender their medicines, which would either be returned on discharge, or destroyed. A new stock was then obtained from the pharmacy and, at discharge, a take-home supply would be requested, with any stock left on the ward being destroyed. This means that each patient could have three sets of medicines; those they brought in, their inpatient medication, and their discharge medication. Moreover, there is a risk that if the medicines that the patient brought in are returned (since they are the patient's property) the patient may take both the original and the discharge sets.

Under one stop dispensing, the newly arrived patient receives a supply of medication in their name which is used for their inpatient stay and, after checking, then forms their take home medication as well. In some cases this supply may be their own medicine, described as 'patients' own drugs'. This requires good policies for checking the medications at admission and discharge.

Reducing risk by proper organization of stock cupboards and drug trolleys

A revision of the Duthie Report by the Royal Pharmaceutical Society of Great Britain (RPSGB, 2005) recommended safety procedures for storing medicines. At the time, the RPSGB was the regulatory body for pharmacy; it has since relinquished this role to the General Pharmaceutical Council (GPhC) but continues (under its new name of the Royal Pharmaceutical Society) as a professional membership body, rather like the RCN. (See Boxes 7.1 and 7.2 for more on the safe storage of medicines.)

All medication must be stored as recommended by the manufacturer. They should be in locked cupboards with separate storage for internal medicines, medicines to be applied externally, medicines for injection,

Box 7.1 Safely storing medicines

- Are they stored in a safe place?
- Are they stored at the correct temperature?
- Who has access to the stored medicines?
- Are keys kept safely?
- Is the medication stored in its original container?
- Who ensures that stocks are maintained?
- Who checks the levels and expiry dates of available stock—particularly of controlled drugs?

Box 7.2 Refrigerating medicines

Medicines in refrigerators should generally be stored between 2° and 8°C. It is not so easy to give a firm rule about the time for which they can be left out of the fridge. Some medication must be refrigerated until it is first used, but then is not returned to the fridge. Most will be kept in the fridge between uses, but some must be brought to room temperature before use and then will not be put back. Generally, the storage conditions are on the manufacturers' packaging, but if in doubt consult a pharmacist for guidance.

controlled drugs and those requiring refrigeration or freezing (Dougherty and Lister, 2008).

> Medicines should be stored at a level of security appropriate to their proposed use and at a level appropriate to the staff present at any time. There is a potential cascade of security levels with the most secure area likely to be the pharmacy, followed by the ward medicine cupboard, medicine trolley, bedside cabinet, and emergency trolley.
>
> RPSGB, 2005, p24.

All healthcare staff have a responsibility to draw attention to unsafe practice with respect to security of medicines. If cupboards are left unlocked, or trolleys are unattended, this should be drawn to the attention of the nurse in charge. It is unacceptable to leave full medicine pots at the patient bedside, which are likely to be unlabelled and perhaps unidentifiable. These pose a risk both to the patient for whom they were

intended and to other patients or visitors such as children who may take them.

The type of container the medicine is supplied in may have been chosen for a specific reason e.g. glyceryl trinitrate tablets must be kept in glass bottles rather than plastic to prevent loss of strength, whilst some tablets that are susceptible to moisture will be in containers with a desiccant in the cap. Care must also be taken to ensure medicines are not stored where there may be fluctuations in temperature. Some medicines must be stored between 2° and 8°C, for which purpose a drugs refrigerator should be used. The maximum and minimum temperatures of such a refrigerator must be monitored and recorded daily. Medicines should never be stored in a refrigerator which is also used for food or drink.

Patients frequently bring their own medicines when they are admitted to hospital and these must also be stored safely and appropriately. You will need to check on your local hospital policy regarding the use and storage of patients' own medicines.

Medicines administration records and record keeping

The NMC (2009) *Guidance on Record Keeping for Nurses and Midwives* (p 1) states that:

> **Good record keeping is an integral part of nursing and midwifery practice, and is essential to the provision of safe and effective care. It is not an optional extra to be fitted in if circumstances allow.**

The responsibility of the pre-registration student is to record the administration of any medicine that they have given to a patient and to have this supervised and countersigned by a registered nurse.

Instructions from a prescriber to administer or supply medicines can be provided in a variety of ways. Within the hospital setting these instructions are often written on a medicines administration record (MAR)—sometimes referred to as drug charts (see Figure 7.1). MARs tend to vary in format from organization to organization, but the basic information that needs to be included on the chart should be the same.

Medication
Administration Record
Care Home Copy

R Refused	**H** Hospitalised	**L** On Leave
S Sleeping	**D** Destroyed	**Q** Not Required
P Pulse Abnormal	**N** Nausea	**O** Other
M Made Available		

MEDICATION	TIME	12/06/2012							19/06/2012							26/06/2012							03/07/2012						
		12	13	14	15	16	17	18	19	20	21	22	23	24	25	26	27	28	29	30	01	02	03	04	05	06	07	08	09
DIPROBASE CREAM PUMP DISP 500G To be applied as directed For external use only Not in Cassette																													

Qty: 0	Received:	By:	Started:	Qty:	Returned by:	Qty:	Destroyed by:

MEDICATION	TIME																												
DORZ'MIDE 2%/TIMOLOL 0.5% EYE 0.2ML Instil ONE drop TWICE a day to both eyes Discard 15 days after opening Not in Cassette	08:00 17:00																												

Qty: 60	Received:	By:	Started:	Qty:	Returned by:	Qty:	Destroyed by:

MEDICATION	TIME																												
LACTULOSE SOLUTION Take THREE 5ML spoonfuls TWICE a day Not in Cassette	08:00 17:00																												

Qty: 0ml	Received:	By:	Started:	Qty:	Returned by:	Qty:	Destroyed by:

MEDICATION	TIME																												
LATANOPROST EYE DROPS 50MCG/ML 2.5ML Instill one drop DAILY to right eye Keep refrigerated. Discard 4 weeks after opening Not in Cassette																													

Qty: 1	Received:	By:	Started:	Qty:	Returned by:	Qty:	Destroyed by:

MEDICATION	TIME																												
LORAZEPAM TABS 1MG Take HALF or ONE tablet when required for agitation. Maximum of TWICE a day. Warning: This medicine may make you sleepy. If this happens, do not drive or use tools or machines. Do not drink alcohol Not in Cassette																													

Qty: 28	Received:	By:	Started:	Qty:	Returned by:	Qty:	Destroyed by:

MEDICATION	TIME																												
OMEPRAZOLE CAPS 20MG Take one at 08:00	08:00/1																												

Qty: 28	Received:	By:	Started:	Qty:	Returned by:	Qty:	Destroyed by:

Figure 7.1 A medicines' administration record. (Patient and practice identifiers have been deleted.)

By definition, an MAR is for a specific, identifiable patient, and it should therefore have information about that patient. Key items of patient information might include:

- Patient name
- Identification number—usually the NHS number, as preferred by NPSA
- Additional identification—for example, a photograph in a long stay setting or a bar code linked to a wristband
- Date of birth/age
- Allergies or contraindications.

There may be other information that is relevant to the area of practice, such as the name and contact details for the doctor/prescribing nurse, home address, and next of kin.

Exercise 7.5

Consider the bullet points. When in practice take time to familiarize yourself with an MAR in your area. Do they contain the medical information in the following list? Are all of the boxes completed? Is there anything missing?

Medical information that needs to be included on an MAR

- The name of the medicine—for example, fluoxetine (NB generic name not trade name, except for some medications where it is important to take the same brand e.g. modified-release diltiazem or theophylline. **There is a list of such medications at the front of the BNF. Check that you can locate it**. For further information on generic and branded drugs please see Chapter 5).
- The strength and form of the medicine to be used e.g. 50 mg capsules, 10 mg/5 ml solution.
- The dose of the medicine—this can be specific or within a range, for example either 20 mg or 20–40 mg as indicated.
- How often the medicine needs to be given (frequency).

- The time interval between doses.
- The maximum daily dose, where appropriate.
- The duration of treatment—for example with antibiotics.
- The route of administration i.e. intramuscular (IM), oral, etc.
- Whether the medicine must be given at a specified time or times or whether it should only be given as required.
- The time of day that the medicine needs to be given.
- If a medicine should be taken before/with/after food.
- Specific requirements e.g. avoiding milk or indigestion remedies for tetracycline, or for alendronic acid—to stand or sit upright for 30 minutes after taking on an empty stomach with plenty of water.
- Other considerations such as patient weight.

MARs must be clearly written and legible. They must be written in ink and must comply with local policy directions.

Exercise 7.6

Where will you make a record of the administration of a medicine?
    Consider what you would do if the patient does not take the medicine.
    Would this make a difference to where you would record this?

For the following scenarios (Case studies 7.1 and 7.2), you may wish to refer to the latest edition of the *BNF* or access the BNF online at: **http://www.bnf.org**
    Return to Chapter 6 if you want to recap the structure of the *BNF*.

Case study 7.1

You are accompanying a registered nurse as they administer metformin 500 mg to Mrs Lucas. You note that this medicine should be given with or after food but Mrs Lucas is refusing her breakfast. What are you going to do and what record will you make? You can find the answer at the end of the chapter.

Case study 7.2

> Mrs Lucas is due to have an operation later that morning. You see in the *BNF* that she should not be given metformin before she has a general anaesthetic, but you have not been given clear instructions about this. What will you do? You can find the answer at the end of the chapter.

What is medicines reconciliation?

Every prescribing decision must be made against a background of the existing medicines being taken. If that information is incorrect or incomplete, the patient may be exposed to unnecessary risk.

Medicines reconciliation is defined by the Institute for Healthcare Improvement (IHI) as the process of obtaining an up-to-date and accurate medication list that has been compared to the most recently available information and has documented any:

- discrepancies
- changes
- deletions
- additions,

resulting in a complete list of medications, accurately communicated. This definition was adopted by the National Prescribing Centre in *Medicines Reconciliation: A guide for implementation* (NPC, 2008). There are some excellent resources for medicines reconciliation on the NPC website at: **http://www.npc.nhs.uk/guidance_mm.php** and on the IHI website: **http://www.ihi.org/knowledge/Pages/ImprovementStories/InnovationatItsBestMedRec.aspx**.

The list of medicines must include all medicines that are actually being taken, whether prescribed or bought. This is not always the same as the list of medicines being prescribed. The patient may be using medicines they have obtained elsewhere, prescribed by someone else or bought; or they may not be taking medication that has been prescribed. While some patients may be reluctant to admit this, it is important that it should be known.

There are particular risks whenever care of a patient passes from one group of professionals to another; on admission to a hospital or care home, on transfer between them, or on discharge from them. It is important that an accurate list of medicines should be transferred with the patient.

Taking a medicines history on admission: the acquisition of necessary practical skills

A comprehensive history should be taken of all medication that the patient is taking. Whereas this is the responsibility of the trained nurse, student nurses might also be involved in gathering this information and a working knowledge of how to take a thorough history is vital for the administration of medicines. This includes the names of prescribed medicines, dosages, routes, and frequency.

Patients frequently cannot remember the names of the medicines that they take but never lead them by making suggestions. Many medicines have similar sounding names and patients may just agree with the suggestion you have given. If the medicines that a patient routinely takes have not been brought into hospital with them then it is wise to ask someone to bring them in for accuracy. Alternatively a trained member of staff might contact the patient's General Practitioner, or their regular pharmacy (if they generally use the same one each time) for information regarding regular medicines.

Patients need to be asked specifically about use of over-the-counter, herbal and homeopathic treatments, dietary supplements, and home remedies (Lilley et al, 2010), as well as illicit drug use. Also remember to ask about eye drops, creams/ointments, and depot injections.

Homeopathic remedies arguably do not interact with conventional medicine, however, it is best practice to elicit a complete picture of substances that a patient is taking, and this will also help the nurse to understand the patient's health beliefs. If the patient's health beliefs are better understood it will be easier for the nurse then to support concordance and adherence.

For more information on patient health beliefs, and on concordance and adherence see Chapter 9.

It is useful to ask direct questions about any hormone preparations as women may not consider oral contraception as 'medication'. Similarly, patients may not volunteer information about health supplements even though these may influence the effectiveness of prescription medicines. For example, kelp may interfere with medicines given to aid thyroid function (UKMi, 2011)

Tobacco use and alcohol intake needs to be recorded as these may affect the effectiveness of prescribed medicines. For example, smoking (Kapoor and Jones, 2005) and chronic alcohol use (Sampson, 1998) may negate the protective skeletal effects of oestrogen replacement therapy. The likely reason for this is that both alcohol and nicotine induce liver enzymes which will cause oestrogen to be metabolized more quickly, reducing the amount of oestrogen available to the tissues. Drinking moderate amounts of alcohol on an occasional basis does not induce these enzymes, which means that this reduced effect is not seen.

An additional example is that smoking decreases levels of the antipsychotic clozapine, so if a patient was unable to smoke while in hospital, the levels of clozapine could increase significantly (Ashir and Petterson, 2008).

Patients should be asked about allergies and any adverse drug reactions (ADR) to medicines in the past, with specific questioning about what the reaction was; this should be clearly recorded in the patient's notes. It is recognized that previous ADR history obtained from hospital patients is often poorly recorded in medical records (Shenfield et al, 2001). Remember, what a patient considers to be an allergic reaction may not actually be a true allergy and may just be a known side effect (Galbraith et al, 2007). For example, the nausea and vomiting associated with some opioids is not actually an allergic reaction but is actually a known side effect and is therefore something that needs to be discussed with the patient. What you are interested in is anyone who reports a previous rash and/or swelling in mouth or throat as a reaction to a substance.

To revise adverse drug reactions please see Chapter 3.

Some patients, including older people or those whose first language is not English, may have relied on someone else to administer their medicines. In this case it is important to gather information from this person as they can help establish a medicines history.

Particular attention needs to be paid to the information gained from patients where it is difficult to ascertain a history regarding their understanding of how to take specific medicines and of the cautions that they might need to be aware of. These include a list of common medicines such as:

1 Steroids

2 Inhalers

3 Insulin

4 Methotrexate

5 Bisphosphonates

6 Lithium

7 Warfarin and other anticoagulants.

Quiz

Can you think why you need to pay particular attention to the medicines listed as 1–7?

To help with your thinking you could try to answer the following questions:

What might they do to the patient?

What are the pharmacokinetics and pharmacodynamics?

What side effects should you look out for?

Who might you need to talk to about the side effects?

What might you need to tell the patient?

You can refer to the latest edition of the *BNF* to help you, or access the *BNF* on line at: **http://www.bnf.org** (free registration required).

Answers at the end of the chapter.

Helping your mentor get a medicines history

Student nurses might be involved in supporting their mentor to gain a medicines history from the patient. As well as asking about medicines history, it is important to acknowledge the significance of age, height, and weight, as these may affect the dosages of medicines. The student needs to be aware that obtaining a thorough medical history is important since this may impact on the medicines prescribed for the patient. For example, the student or their mentor may need to ask the patient about any cardiovascular, renal, or hepatic disease, as this may affect the medicines prescribed and the dosages given. The patient might want to know why you are asking all of these questions.

Exercise 7.7

Think about the questions that need to be asked by the nurse when gaining a medicines history. Consider how you would communicate with the patient when asking these questions. What questions might the patient ask and how could you answer these? Some are listed here. You might want to discuss this with your mentor.

Some examples of questions a patient might ask:

- How do I take the medicine?
- Why do I need to take it before, with, or after food?
- What will the medicine do to me?
- What side effects might I expect?
- Why can't I drink alcohol when taking this medicine?
- How many days do I need to take the medicine for before it starts to work?
- What do I do if the medicine does not work?
- What do I do if I cannot tolerate the medicine?
- Can I cut this patch in half to save money on the prescription?
- How long will I need to take the medicine for?
- Can I crush this tablet if as it is hard to swallow?
- Can I cut the tablet in half?
- Can I take it as a syrup instead?

What other questions did you come up with? Refer to the section of pharmacokinetics in Chapter 3 for more ideas.

National standards for medicines management

The national service framework for older people (DH, 2001a)

Although older people are not the only ones who are taking medicines and who might be at risk as a result of mismanagement of their medicines, the older population is living longer and so are the numbers of medicines that they are taking (see Chapter 5). The National Service Framework for Older people sets the standard for medicines management in this age group. It recognizes medicines management as being, 'a fundamental component of each of the NSF standards', (DH, 2001a, p 12).

The supportive booklet *Medicines and Older People* (DH, 2001b) can be accessed by clicking on the following link: **http://www.dh.gov.uk/prod_consum_dh/groups/dh_digitalassets/@dh/@en/documents/digitalasset/dh_4067247.pdf**.

The executive summary of the KSF can be found by clicking on the following link: **http://www.dh.gov.uk/prod_consum_dh/groups/dh_digitalassets/@dh/@en/documents/digitalasset/dh_4058295.pdf**.

Key points highlighted in the NSF executive summary (DH, 2001a) that relate to medicines management are listed:

- Many adverse reactions to medicines could be prevented.
- Some medicines are under-used in older people.
- Medicines may not be taken as intended.
- Repeat prescriptions may result in waste.
- Poor communication between hospitals and primary care can mean changes to medication or lack of information about an older person's medication.
- Poor information on the medicine label.
- Access to the GP surgery or pharmacy can be a problem.
- A carer's potential contribution and needs are often not addressed.

(DH, 2001c, p 23).

In *Medicines and Older People* (DH, 2001b) a number of ways are suggested in which registered nurses are involved in supporting the NSF standards. Nurses in primary care conducting health checks for patients over 75-years-old can screen for medicine-related problems and bring them to the attention of the GP or pharmacist. A proportion of them may become nurse consultants or specialist nurses, in which role they may be non-medical prescribers. Even if they are not, they can be sources of excellent medicines advice for their patients. Nurses can also assess and assist adherence to medicines, perhaps suggesting adjustments that can be made to aid patients such as diary cards or electronic pill reminders. Some practice nurses run clinics for patients with long-term conditions where the elderly will be well represented.

In the same way the Department of Health have produced *The National Service Framework for Children and Young People* and standard 10 is entitled: Medicines for children and young people (DH, 2004b). The standard calls for a safe and child centred approach to medicines management for children. It requires medicines to be easy for children to use and that they are given in partnership with the child and carers, taking into account children who might be disadvantaged and those who have multiple needs and who might be taking multiple medicines.

The main themes related to safety in standard 10 are listed here:

- Dose, volume, and rate calculations are carefully checked and recorded,

- The child's age, weight, and dose is included on prescriptions,

- A child's allergies should be recorded clearly,

- Oral syringes are used to give liquid medicines, especially for babies and younger children.

This standard can be accessed by following this link: **http://www.dh.gov.uk/en/Publicationsand-statistics/Publications/PublicationsPolicyAnd-Guidance/Browsable/DH_4870567**.

Reflection point

Consider the bullet points quoted from both lists of standards (older people and children). You might wish to reflect on a patient you have nursed who has been affected by some of these themes. How could nursing interventions have prevented some of these concerns from happening?

The role of the Care Quality Commission

It is likely that as you progress through your training you will experience working in a variety of public and private settings. Care and clinical governance within the private sector and in hospitals that are not Foundation Trusts are monitored by the Care Quality Commission (CQC), which incorporates the former Commission for Social Care Inspection (CSCI). The CQC sets minimum standards and measures and monitors the quality of care that is provided for all people who are dependent on care, either within the NHS in hospitals or in other care organizations and settings. It provides advice for professionals who are administering medicines within care homes. The remit of CQC is changing over the next few years and it will be useful to check their website periodically to see these changes developing: **http://www.cqc.org.uk**

A set of national minimum standards was produced by their predecessors CSCI in conjunction with the Department of Health in 2001(d) and 2003. Regulation 13 (2) of the *Care Homes* regulations (DH, 2003) stated that 'a registered professional must make arrangements for the . . . safe administration . . . of medicines prescribed for the people they care for'. The standards acknowledge that where possible people should be encouraged to self-administer their medicines. This ethos is also supported by the NMC (2008). However, self-administration is not always possible and both the CQC and NMC have built robust guidance into their mandatory standards to support registered health professionals to administer medicines to patients and to delegate this administration to designated and appropriately trained staff who have been assessed as being competent to do so.

Registered health professionals and students who are working in nursing homes and care homes in both the private and NHS setting must make sure that they are familiar with and adhere to these standards and must be aware that they work within their professional codes of conduct (NMC, 2008) and adhere to the NMC (2010) standards for medicines management.

Summary

This chapter has revised the accountability and responsibilities of the student and trained nurse in relation to medicines management. We have looked at:

- The necessity for safe systems, policies, and procedures, and explained that nurses need to understand these,
- The key standards and national drivers that support nurses to be involved in the safe management of medicines,
- The responsibilities and accountabilities of the nurse in relation to these drivers.

For more information regarding the responsibilities and accountability of the nurse please see Chapters 1 and 10.

Further reading

Institute for Healthcare Improvement. For resources to assist in medicines reconciliation, see: http://www.ihi.org/IHI/Topics/PatientSafety/MedicationSystems/ (accessed 26 May 2012).

National Prescribing Centre (NPC) Introduction to Medicines Management e Learning available at: http://www.npc.nhs.uk/developing_systems/intro/index.php (accessed 25 May 2012).

NPC e Learning for Medicines Reconciliation with Case Studies available at: http://www.npc.nhs.uk/improving_safety/medicines_reconciliation/index.php (accessed 25 May 2012).

References

Ashir M, and Petterson L (2008). Smoking bans and clozapine levels. Advances in Psychiatric Treatment 14; 398–399

BNF see Joint Formulary Committee.

Department of Health (2001a), The National Service Framework for Older People. London: TSO.

Department of Health (2001b), Medicines and older people implementing medicines-related aspects of the NSF for older people. London: TSO.

Department of Health (2001c), The National Service Framework for Older People. London: TSO.

Department of Health (2001d), Care Homes for Older People. National Minimum Standards and the Care Homes Regulations 2001. London:TSO.

Department of Health (2003), Care Homes for Adults (18–65) and Supplementary Standards for Care Homes Accommodating Young People Aged 16 and 17 National Minimum Standards Care Homes Regulations February 2003. London: TSO.

Department of Health (2004a), Management of Medicines—a resource to support implementation of the wider aspects of medicines management for the National Service Frameworks for Diabetes, Renal Services and Long-Term Conditions. London: TSO Available at: http://www.dh.gov.uk/prod_consum_dh/groups/dh_digitalassets/@dh/@en/documents/digitalasset/dh_4088755.pdf (accessed 26 May 2012).

Department of Health (2004b), The National Service Framework for Children and Young People. London: TSO.

Department of Health (2006), Medicines Matters. A Guide to Mechanisms for the Prescribing, Supply and Administration of Medicines. London: TSO.

Dougherty L, and Lister S (eds.) (2008), The Royal Marsden Hospital Manual of Clinical Nursing Procedures. Oxford: Wiley-Blackwell.

Elliott M, and Liu Y (2010). The nine rights of medication administration: an overview, British Journal of Nursing, 19; 300–305.

Galbraith A, Bullock S, Manias E, Hunt B and Richards A (2007), Fundamentals of Pharmacology. An applied approach for nursing and health (2nd ed). Harlow: Pearson Education Ltd.

Joint Formulary Committee (2012). British National Formulary (64th ed). London: BMJ Group and Pharmaceutical Press.

Kapoor D, and Jones TH (2005). Smoking and hormones in health and endocrine disorders, European Journal of Endocrinology, 152; 491–499.

Lilley LL, Collins SR, Harrington S, and Snyder JS (2010), Pharmacology and the Nursing Process, (6th ed). Mosby: St Louis.

National Audit Office (2007), *Prescribing Costs in Primary Care. Report by the Comptroller and Auditor General. HC 454 Session 2006-2007. 18 May 2007*: http://www.publications.parliament.uk/pa/cm200708/cmselect/cmpubacc/173/173.pdf (accessed 26th May 2012).

National Patient Safety Agency (2004), *Seven Steps to Patient Safety: Full Reference Guide*. Available at: http://www.nrls.npsa.nhs.uk/resources/collections/seven-steps-to-patient-safety/?entryid45=59787 (accessed 24 May 2012).

National Patient Safety Agency (2009), *Safety in Doses. Improving the Use of Medicines in the NHS. Learning from National Reporting 2007*. London: National Reporting and Learning Service, NPSA.

National Prescribing Centre (2002), *Modernising Medicines Management: A guide to achieving benefits for patients, professionals and the NHS*, Liverpool: NPC, available at: http://www.npc.nhs.uk/developing_systems/intro/resources/library_good_practice_guide_mmmbook1_2002.pdf (accessed 25 May 2012).

National Prescribing Centre (2008), *Medicines Reconciliation: A guide for implementation*, available at: http://www.npc.nhs.uk/improving_safety/medicines_reconciliation/resources/reconciliation_guide.pdf (accessed 26 May 2012).

Nursing and Midwifery Council (2008), *The Code: Standards of Conduct, Performance and Ethics for Nurses and Midwives*. London: NMC.

Nursing and Midwifery Council (2009), *Guidance on Record Keeping for Nurses and Midwives*. London: NMC.

Nursing and Midwifery Council (2010), *Standards for Medicines Management*. London: NMC.

The Royal Pharmaceutical Society of Great Britain (RPSGB) (2005), *The safe and secure handling of medicines: a team approach (A revision of the Duthie Report (1988) led by the Hospital Pharmacists' Group of the Royal Pharmaceutical Society)*. Available at: http://www.rpharms.com/support-pdfs/safsechandmeds.pdf (accessed on 24 May 2012).

Sampson HW (1998). Alcohol's harmful effects on bone. *Alcohol Health and Research World*, 22; 190–194.

Shenfield G, Robb T, and Duguid M (2001). Recording previous adverse drug reactions—a gap in the system, *British Journal of Clinical Pharmacology*,51; 623-626

Trueman P, Taylor D, Lowson K, Newbould J, Blighe A, Bury M, et al (2010), Evaluation of the Scale, Causes and Costs of Waste Medicines, York Health Economics Consortium and The School of Pharmacy, University of London, for the Department of Health, available at: http://php.york.ac.uk/inst/yhec/web/news/documents/Evaluation_of_NHS_Medicines_Waste_Nov_2010.pdf (accessed 7 June 2012).

UKMi (2011), Can patients on levothyroxine take sea kelp? Available at: http://www.nelm.nhs.uk/en/NeLM-Area/Evidence/Medicines-Q--A/Can-patients-on-levothyroxine-take-sea-kelp/?query=kelpandrank=100 (accessed 7 June 2012).

Vreven R, and De Kock M (2005). Metformin lactic acidosis and anaesthesia: myth or reality? *Acta Anaesthesiologica Belgica*, 56; 297–302.

Answers to case study questions

Case study 7.1

You will need to discuss this with the nurse responsible for the administration but recognize that you need to be clear about what is appropriate if you accept the delegated responsibility for administration. Metformin can be given with a very small amount of food so you may be able to persuade Mrs Lucas to eat just a little. If not then you will need to report this and ensure that it is clearly documented.

Follow up questions: consider how you might then act if Mrs Lucas still refuses. Who else might you involve? You might wish to discuss this with your mentor.

Case study 7.2

The operation may not require general anaesthetic, but if it does, it may have to be postponed if Mrs Lucas has been given metformin. At the very least, you should raise the matter with the nurse in charge before giving the dose.

The reason for stopping metformin is that it is associated with lactic acidosis, a life-threatening condition in which lactic acid collects in the blood. The risk that this will happen is increased by surgery, although no cause for this has been proven (Vreven and De Kock, 2005). However, many surgeons and anaesthetists prefer to suspend metformin until the patient's biochemistry returns to normal after surgery.

Quiz answers

These medicines need special attention because:

1 **Steroids:** If a patient has been taking regular doses of steroids and needs to stop taking them, the dose must be gradually reduced. An abrupt withdrawal of steroids could lead to anaphylactic shock (see latest version of

BNF). Some individuals with conditions such as chronic obstructive pulmonary disease (COPD) or asthma may take short courses of oral steroids and accuracy about this is important. There is a risk that the adrenal glands will be suppressed by long-term or frequent, repeated short courses of steroids so the trained nurse would want to know when they last took any, the dosage and for how long they were taken. If the patient has taken more than 40 mg prednisolone (or its equivalent) for more than a week, or any dose for more than 3 weeks, or repeated short courses, the steroid should be withdrawn slowly. This is described in detail in BNF section 6.3.2. Patients taking long-term steroids, either orally or as inhalers, should carry a steroid card—this may provide useful information to the nurse or in the case of an emergency admission.

2 **Inhalers:** Patients usually know the colour of their inhalers but may not know the name. Beware of making assumptions when they describe the colour. For example, a 'green inhaler' may be Serevent® or Atrovent®. Different types of inhaler are used and it is important to know which type the patient uses.

3 **Insulin:** There is a need to gain information on the brand of insulin used, the device for administration and the dosages used at the present time.
This is evidenced by the regular National Diabetes Inpatient Audits (NaDIA) undertaken by NHS Diabetes. The reports of these audits are accessible at: **http://www.diabetes.nhs.uk/information_and_data/ diabetes_audits/national_diabetes_inpatient_ audit/**.
The 2010 audit included the following findings:
37.1% of inpatients with diabetes experienced at least one medication error,
26.0% of charts had prescription errors and 20.0% had one or more medication management errors,
Patients with medication errors had twice the rate of severe hypoglycaemia (18.1% vs. 7.9%).
Many of these errors involved the patient being given an insulin other than the one they have been using, or in a device that they have not been trained to use.
The dose given at the last injection was not always clear.

4 **Methotrexate** is recognized as a high-risk drug by the National Patient Safety Agency. It can potentially cause bone marrow suppression preventing the manufacture of white blood cells. This can be fatal. The risk is reduced if the patient takes a weekly dose rather than daily doses, and the gastrointestinal side-effects of

methotrexate are reduced if folic acid is given after the methotrexate (but not on the same day). The days on which methotrexate and folic acid are given should therefore be noted to ensure that the patient can be given it on the correct day.

5 **Biphosphonates:** Many older patients take bisphosphonates and again these are often taken weekly so the day they take them must be noted. There are very specific instructions for taking these tablets and this is a good opportunity to check patients are taking their medicines correctly. See details at: **http:// www.nyrdtc.nhs.uk/docs/smu/RDTC%20SMU%20 Bis%20v1.pdf**.

6 **Lithium** is used in the prophylaxis and treatment of a range of mental health conditions. There is little difference between the levels needed for therapeutic effect and those at which the patient may suffer toxicity. Overdosage can be fatal. It is therefore vital that the patient adheres to their treatment plan and that the levels of lithium in their plasma are monitored regularly. Failure to attend for monitoring or abrupt discontinuation of lithium could be dangerous. There are a number of brands, and patients should not be moved between brands once stabilized except under careful supervision. NPSA guidance on lithium can be found at: **http:// www.npsa.nhs.uk/corporate/news/close-monitoring-of-patients-prescribed-lithium-will-reduce-harm/?locale=en**.

7 **Warfarin and other anticoagulants** are used to reduce the risk of blood clots, but they also increase the risk of haemorrhage. It is therefore vital that the ability of the blood to clot (measured as the International Normalised Ratio or INR) is regularly checked to ensure that the doses given are optimal. There is a complication in that warfarin is extensively bound to protein, so it interacts readily with a wide range of medicines with very different uses that also bind to plasma proteins. For safety reasons, healthcare professionals should ensure that the patient is using the latest prescription instructions and is being regularly monitored. Nurses will also be alert for any signs of bleeding that, perhaps, the patient may not see. Prescriptions for warfarin frequently have minimal dosage information, because it changes according to need, so it is likely that tablet containers will not have a dose on them – and even if they do, it should be checked against the treatment chart or care plan. Patients should have a 'Yellow Book', which is a patient-held record of their dosage and monitoring results.

8 Medicines Management: Drug Calculations

CHAPTER CONTENTS

- Introduction to drug calculations
- SI units
- How to convert metric units

- Calculating drug dosages
- Weight-related doses
- Summary

LEARNING OUTCOMES

After reading this chapter you should be able to:

- Understand the importance of drug calculations
- Recognize different types of calculations
- Know where you can find help with numeracy
- Successfully complete basic calculations for medicines.

Introduction to drug calculations

Are you good at drug calculations? This is a question you must ask yourself and be honest about the answer. There is no room for inaccuracies when calculating medicine dosages and if you are not happy working with numbers then you need to practise.

Drug calculation is a critical area when managing medicines and is open to error. All health professionals who are dispensing, supplying, or administering drugs will need to perform drug calculations to a greater or lesser extent. Registered professionals are accountable and responsible for their decisions and actions and cannot rely on others to check the accuracy of their calculations.

The NMC's medicines management skills cluster for pre-registration nursing programmes (2010) states that patients can trust registered nurses to undertake medicines calculations correctly and safely. Numeracy skills are required to ensure this and to enable registered nurses to perform the drug calculations required to administer medicines safely via appropriate routes. All branches of nursing must also recognize the specific requirements for children and other groups with regard to medicines' calculations.

Within this chapter we offer some explanations and the chance to practise some calculations. There is an expectation that all pre-registration health care professionals will have at least GCSE mathematics or equivalent, such as the Scottish Certificate of Education, therefore explanations will assume you have this level of knowledge. Universities recognize that some students have real difficulty with numeracy and they make additional support available from local study skill centres. Your personal tutor will have details.

SI units

One area of frequent confusion is the use of SI units (International System of Units). SI units are units of measurement for example grams, milligrams, or micrograms, which measure weight; and millilitres or litres, which measure volume. When calculating drug doses, make sure that you are aware of the SI unit that is being used, for example, grams or milligrams, litres or millilitres; see Table 8.1 for equivalences of weight and volume.

The recommendation is that, within medicines management, decimals should be avoided whenever possible. For example, 500 mg should be used instead of 0.5 g, and 125 mcg (micrograms) rather than 0.125 mg. Similarly using the terminal zero following a decimal point (as in 1.0 mg) should be avoided. Of course, the last zero must be kept if it is before the decimal point—there is a difference between 10 and 1! The word microgram should be written in full whenever possible to avoid confusion between mcg or µg (abbreviations for microgram) and mg (milligram). Box 8.1 shows some of the common abbreviations used for SI units you are likely to come across when performing drug calculations.

How to convert metric units

Converting a number from one metric unit to another involves moving the decimal place to the left or the right. To work out how many decimal places to move:

1 Identify the amount to be converted

2 Note the metric units

Box 8.1 Abbreviations for SI units

> mcg or µg = micrograms
> mg = milligrams
> g = grams
> µl or mcl = microlitres
> mL or ml = millilitres
> l = litres

The abbreviation for litres is often given in upper case, as in mL or L. Both upper and lower case are used, but whichever we pick, we should be consistent. Originally lower case was used, but to reduce the risk of confusion between the letter l or the number 1, some authorities suggest using the capital L.

3 Count how many times must you multiply or divide by 10 to convert one unit to the other (this will tell you how many places to move the decimal point)

4 Move the decimal point the number of places from the given unit to the desired unit (see Box 8.2).

Example

Convert 5 grams to milligrams.

1 Identify the amount to be converted:
   5 grams to milligrams

2 Note the metric units: **grams** and **milligrams** (Remember 1 gram = 1000 milligrams)

3 How many times must you multiply or divide by 10 to convert grams to milligrams?
   1 to 1000—i.e. three zeros more

4 Move the decimal point this number of places to convert from the given unit to the desired unit:
   If 5 is rewritten with several zeros after the decimal point then: **5.000 → 50.00 → 500.0 → 5000**

   Therefore **5 grams is the same as 5000 milligrams**. (The decimal place is moved 3 places to the right.)

Table 8.1 Equivalences of weight and volume.

Units of measurement (SI units) for weight	Units of measurement (SI units) for volume
1000 micrograms = 1 milligram	1000 microlitres = 1 millilitre
1000 milligrams = 1 gram	1000 millilitres = 1 litre

As a check that you have moved the decimal point the right way, remember that milligrams are much smaller than grams so there should be more of them!

If you were converting 25 grams to milligrams then move the decimal point 3 places to the right = 25000 milligrams (three more zeros).

Example

Now convert 7500 milligrams to grams.

1 Identify the amount to be converted:
   7500 milligrams to **grams**

2 Note the metric units: **milligrams** and **grams**
   (Remember 1000 milligrams = 1 gram)

3 How many times must you multiply or divide by 10 to convert milligrams to grams?
   1000 to 1—i.e. three zeros less

4 Move the decimal point the number of places from the given unit to the desired unit.
   7500 → 750 → 75 → 7.5
   Therefore **7500 milligrams is the same as 7.5 grams**. (The decimal place is moved 3 places to the left.)

To check that you have moved the decimal point the right way, remember that grams are much bigger than milligrams so there should be fewer of them!

If you were converting 25000 milligrams to grams then move the decimal point 3 places to the left = 25 grams (three zeros less).

If you want to practise try the examples in Exercise 8.1.

Box 8.2 Remember these simple rules

When you change from big units to smaller units the decimal point moves to the right.
   When you change from small units to bigger units the decimal point moves to the left.

Exercise 8.1

1 Convert 65 000 milligrams into grams
2 Convert 78 grams into milligrams
3 Convert 3.5 grams into milligrams.

Did you manage to get them right? You can find the answers at the end of the chapter.

Common mistakes in drug calculations

The main areas of error when calculating drug dosages include:

● Moving the decimal point in the wrong direction when converting dosages to the same units of measurement (SI units) for example grams to milligrams or litres to millilitres
● Miscalculating quantities of tablets/dressings etc. to be administered over a period of time
● Miscalculating time interval between doses
● Miscalculating volume of drug in solution
● Miscalculating the rate of administration (intravenous fluid).

The remainder of this chapter will show how these mistakes can be avoided and give you the opportunity to practise your learning.

Calculating drug dosages

Solutions

For a dose that is in a solution ensure that the dosage of the drug is the same level of SI unit as the solution that it is in. If this is not the case then convert it so that it is.

Example

You have 0.005 grams in 10 millilitres but these are not the same level of SI unit (remember Table 8.1).

0.005 **grams** in 10 millilitres is better expressed as 5 **milligrams** in 10 millilitres (5 mg in 10 mL).

Tablets

Moving on to some common calculations required in clinical practice, you will find that there are some straightforward formulae that will help. We will start with calculations for tablets.

Calculating the number of tablets to be given as a single dose

The formula to use is:

required dose / stock dose = amount to be administered

Example

Mr Gregory has been prescribed 60 mg of codeine phosphate to be administered 4-hourly. The available stock dose (the dose in which the tablets are supplied) is 30 mg. How many tablets will you need to give for a single dose?

60 mg (required dose) / 30 mg (stock dose) = 2 (amount to be administered)For a single dose Mr Gregory will require 2 tablets.

Calculating the number of tablets to be administered over a period of time

This is particularly important when planning a patient's discharge to ensure sufficient supplies to complete a course of antibiotics for example. It is also important to check that medicines have been prescribed in the form that is most acceptable for the patient as this will support adherence. For example, a single 1 gram tablet might be more acceptable for the patient to take than two 500 milligram tablets; or an oral solution might be more acceptable in the case of a patient who has difficulty in swallowing tablets.

When calculating the number of tablets to be given in 24 hours you will need to be aware of the time interval between the doses, for example, to be given 4-hourly. You will also need to be aware of the dose of the drug to be given and the stock dose of the drug.

To calculate the total number of tablets needing to be prescribed over a time period:

- Identify the dose of the tablet that is required to be given
- Identify the strength of the stock dose of the tablet (what dose does it come in?)
- Identify the total number of tablets to be given as a single dose
- Identify the time interval between dosages

- Identify the number of times that you need to give the dose in one day and therefore the number of tablets required for one day
- If tablets are to be given no less than 4-hourly for a maximum period of 24 hours then you must divide the required time period for the total dose to have been given (in this case 24 hours) by the time interval between doses (in this case not less than every 4 hours)

24 / 4 = 6

- The tablets therefore need to be given six times a day with an interval of not less than 4 hours between administrations
- Identify then the total number of tablets required for the total number of days they must be taken.

Example

Let's return to Mr Gregory who has been prescribed 60 mg of codeine phosphate to be administered 4-hourly for 24 hours.

Required single dose of 60 mg.

The available stock dose (the dose in which the tablets are supplied) of codeine phosphate is 30 mg.

To give 60 mg for each dose you will need to two 30 mg tablets every four hours.

The time interval between doses is 4 hours.

The number of times that the dose needs to be given in 24 hours is calculated by dividing the total number of hours by the minimum dose frequency. In this case:

24 / 4 = 6 (6 doses needed in 24 hours).

To work out the total dose multiply the dose given at each single administration by the dose frequency (how many times the dose is given in 24 hours).

60 mg x 6 times in 24 hours = total dose in 24 hours = 360 mg.

To work out the number of tablets to be prescribed for a 24-hour period multiply the number of tablets to be given at each dose by the number of times to be given in 24 hours.

2 tablets (at each single administration) × 6 (times a day) = 12 tablets to be prescribed for a 24-hour period.

Mr Gregory should be taking 12 tablets in 24 hours.

Calculating the total number of tablets to be given for longer than 24 hours

Multiply the number of tablets to be given over a 24-hour period by the number of days that the tablets are to be given for.

Example

We will continue with Mr Gregory's tablets. He is now going to need enough tablets to continue taking them for 5 days. See Table 8.2.

12 tablets to be given in 24 hours (1 day)

Number of tablets to be prescribed for 5 days = 12 × 5 = 60 tablets.

Checking that patients have the required number of tablets can help ensure courses of treatment are continued or completed appropriately.

Liquid drugs administered orally or by injection

Now we will move on to calculations for liquids, using the same formula as for calculating dosages for tablets.

Remember that the prescribed dose must be in the same SI unit as the stock dose.

Example

In this example the SI unit of the prescribed dose is the same as the stock dose.

To administer 20 mg of methylprednisolone acetate when the stock strength is 40 mg in 1mL, how many millilitres will you administer?

The formula to use is:

required dose / stock dose = volume to be administered

The numbers are now placed in the formula:

$$20 / 40 = 2 / 4 = 1 / 2 \text{ or } 0.5$$

What you must remember here is that the 40 mg is in 1 mL so 2 / 4 or 1 / 2 of 1 mL is the amount to administer.

$$1 / 2 \text{ mL} = 0.5 \text{ mL}$$

Therefore 0.5 mL is the amount to administer.

Exercise 8.2 Calculating liquid drug dosages

Now try calculating this one on your own: if there is 40 mg of the drug in 5 mL what is the amount you would need to administer to give a dose of 20 mg?
You can find the answer at the end of the chapter.

Ointments

% w/v is a way of describing the percentage mass (weight) of the drug in a given volume of ointment. It is expressed as the number of grams per 100 mL.

% w/w is a similar way of expressing the percentage, but in this case it is the mass of an ingredient per 100 g of the ointment or cream.

Table 8.2 Calculating Mr Gregory's tablets: the table shows the number of tablets for each dose on each day.

	1st dose	2nd dose	3rd dose	4th dose	5th dose	6th dose
Day 1	2	2	2	2	2	2
Day 2	2	2	2	2	2	2
Day 3	2	2	2	2	2	2
Day 4	2	2	2	2	2	2
Day 5	2	2	2	2	2	2
Total for each day	10	10	10	10	10	10
Total for course	60 tablets					

Example

An ointment containing 8% w/v = 8 g of the drug in 100 mL of the solution or ointment base. So, firstly, what must we do?

How many grams of the drug in 1 mL?

$$8 / 100 = 0.08$$

so there are 0.08 g in 1 mL.

Then to make the SI units the same level we need to move the decimal point 3 places to the right.

$$0.08 \text{ g} = 80 \text{ mg}$$

Therefore, there are 80mg of the drug in 1 mL of ointment.

Intravenous infusions

Giving sets are commonly designed to administer fluid at either 20 drops per mL or 60 drops per ml (as a micro drip).

To calculate the number of drops to be given per mL:

Rate (drops / min) = volume (drops) / time (minutes).

Example

1000 mL is to be given over 10 hours, and the giving set delivers 20 drops per mL.

Rate = volume (drops) / time (hours) × 60
   = 1000 mLx 20 drops/mL/ 10 hours × 60
   = 20000 / 600 = 33.3 drops per minute.

This is not practical to administer therefore you would need to make it into a whole number by rounding down to 33. (We round down if the figure following the whole number is less than 5 and we round up if it is larger.)

Weight-related doses

Sometimes, especially in paediatrics, we have to give a dose related to the patient's weight. For example, the dose of cetirizine for a child of 1–2 years in given in the *BNF for Children* as 250 micrograms/kg twice daily, and the available liquid medicine contains 5 mg cetirizine in each 5 mL.

Example

For a child of 8 kg, what dose—and therefore what volume of solution—would you give?

If each kg requires 250 micrograms, then:

8 kg will need 8 × 250 micrograms = 2000 micrograms.
2000 micrograms = 2 milligrams.

The available solution is 5 mg/5 mL, which is the same as 1mg in 1mL.

Thus, if we need 2 milligrams, we will need 2mL of solution.

Exercise 8.3 allows you to practice drug calculations.

Exercise 8.3 End of chapter exercise

You are conducting a medicines round on a ward in a community hospital. You have another nurse to check your sums but you must calculate independently and then compare your answers.

In one four-bedded bay you greet Mrs Green. Mrs Green was prescribed erythromycin tablets 250 mg four times a day for 7 days and has taken them for 2 days. Now she is going home. How many tablets will she need to be given to complete the course?

Next to Mrs Green is Mrs Gold. Mrs Gold has been prescribed 62.5 micrograms of digoxin each morning but she cannot swallow tablets. The digoxin elixir you have contains 50 micrograms/mL. How many millilitres will you need to give her?

Opposite Mrs Gold is Miss Brown. Miss Brown has been having 5 mg morphine sulphate every four hours to combat her pain. Now the doctor intends to use a syringe driver and has asked you to ensure that the ward has enough stock of morphine sulphate to fill the driver for 24 hours at the rate of 5 mg per 4 hours. How much will you need?

Miss Brown's neighbour is Ms Violet. Ms Violet has been prescribed gentamicin by injection at a dose of 5 mg/kg daily, divided into three equal doses. She weighs 60 kg. How much should be given at each dose?

You will find the answers at the end of the chapter.

Summary

This chapter has provided details and examples to help you develop your skills and:

- Understand the importance of drug calculations
- Recognize different types of calculations
- Know where you can find help with numeracy
- Successfully complete basic calculations for medicines.

Further reading

There are a number of textbooks available to help with numeracy. Examples include:

Lapham R and Agar H (2009) Drug calculations for nurses: A Step-by-step Approach (3rd ed). London: Hodder Arnold.

Gatsford JD, and Phillips N (2006), Nursing calculations. London: Churchill Livingstone.

A more advanced text is:

Rees J, Smith I, and Smith B (2004), *Introduction to pharmaceutical calculations*. London: Pharmaceutical Press.

Ian Smith and Judith Rees have produced a companion volume which is useful for testing knowledge *Pharmaceutical Calculations Workbook* (2005).

A recent primer on general numeracy techniques which is particularly helpful if you need support with your arithmetical skills:

Shihab P (2009) *Numeracy in nursing and healthcare: calculations and practice*. London: Pearson.Useful websites: http://www.bbc.co.uk/skillswise/numbers http://www.bbc.co.uk/schools/ks2bitesize/maths

References

Nursing and Midwifery Council (2010) *Essential Skills Clusters (ESC) for Pre-registration Nursing Programmes*. Available at: http://standards.nmc-uk.org/Published-Documents/Standards%20for%20pre-registration%20nursing%20education%2016082010.pdf (accessed 24 May 2012).

Paediatric Formulary Committee (2012), *BNF for Children* (2012–2013). London: BMJ Group, Pharmaceutical Press, and RCPCH Publications.

Answers

Exercise 8.1

Converting SI units

1 65 000 milligrams = 65 grams
2 78 grams = 78 000 milligrams
3 3.5 grams = 3500 milligrams

Exercise 8.2

Calculating liquid drug dosages

We have already worked out that the proportion necessary is 0.5 of what we have. When this was 1 mL it was straightforward. Now we need to remember that we have a stock dose of 40 mg in 5 mL.

$$5 \text{ mL} / 2 = 2.5 \text{ mL}$$

Exercise 8.3

Mrs Green

Mrs Green was prescribed a 7 day course and has taken 2 days, so she needs 5 days' treatment. She takes 4 tablets a day, so she will need 20 tablets.

Mrs Gold

Using the formula

required dose / stock dose × what it's in (the stock volume)

Mrs Gold needs:

62.5 × 1 mL / 50 = 1.25 mL of the digoxin elixir.

Miss Brown

The number of 4-hour intervals in 24 hours is 24 / 4 = 6; so Miss Brown has had six doses a day, each of 5 mg, so she will need 30 mg (5 mg × 6) morphine sulphate for the next 24 hours.

Ms Violet

Ms Violet needs 5 mg/kg of gentamicin and weighs 60 kg, so in total she needs 60 × 5 mg = 300 mg. When this is divided into three equal doses, each will contain 100 mg.

9 The Nurse's Role in Promoting Concordance

CHAPTER CONTENTS

- Compliance versus adherence and concordance
- Things that can go wrong with medication
- Concordance
- Patient health: beliefs and concordance
- Adherence
- Adverse drug reactions and concordance
- Patients posing particular difficulty
- Preparing a patient for discharge
- Expert patient programme
- Summary

LEARNING OUTCOMES

- To support an understanding of the theory of **concordance**
- Working in partnership with your patient, to relate this knowledge to the achievement of concordance in the consultation process.

Compliance versus adherence and concordance

The NMC code states that when caring for your patient: you must work with others to protect and promote the health and wellbeing of those in your care, their families and carers, and the wider community (NMC, 2008). In the past, nurses would give medicines to patients, and the patients would usually do as they were told and take the medicine without questioning the doctor or health professional. The word used to explain this interaction in the world of medicines management is compliance.

This term originates from a traditional biomedical model of care where the patient is viewed as a list of symptoms and it implies that in the act of giving medicines nurses were doing something active to treat the patient's illness and symptoms. It also implies that the patient was receiving medicines from the nurse; the act of receiving is a passive concept whereby the patient is having something done to them. If they passively followed the instructions that they had been given and took their medicines correctly, then they would get better.

What's wrong with compliance?

The traditional biomedical model of compliance has not proved very effective in terms of patient treatment. If the patient is not given reasons why their treatment is important, or feels that they have not been involved in the decision, the common result is non-compliance. Sometimes this is intentional (the patient decides not to take their medication), and sometimes unintentional (the patient does not know what they need to take, or when). This has cost implications for the National Health Service. If prescribed drugs, often paid for by the NHS, remain unused the patient's illness may not improve, resulting in the supply of another prescription (or other treatment) that might have been avoided if they had taken the medicine which was initially prescribed. Indeed the World Health Organization identified that less than 50% of patients adhere to their medicines' regimens (WHO 2003). An American study identified that 33–69% of hospital admissions with ensuing expense to health care delivery are due to poor adherence to medication (Osterberg and Blaschke, 2005).

Things that can go wrong with medication

- Patients may be given the wrong drug by the health professional
- Patients who are self-administering might have been supplied with the correct drug but might mistakenly take a different one
- Patients might take the wrong dose
- Patients may take the medication at the wrong time of day
- Patients may forget to take the drug
- Patients may choose not to take the drug and might not tell the health professional
- The patient might not understand what is being said to them.

Exercise 9.1

Can you think of other things that might go wrong with medication? Make a list.

Concordance

Concordance involves a new approach to prescribing and taking medicines based on partnership. Instead of patients being expected to 'do as they are told', they are invited to agree on the treatment that they are going to take. The patient and health care professional participate as partners to reach an agreement on the illness and treatment. Their agreement draws on the experiences, beliefs, and wishes of the patient to decide when, how, and why to use medicines and therefore should respect patient autonomy (the right to make decisions for themselves). Healthcare professionals should treat one another as partners and recognize each other's skills to improve the patient's participation. Concordance requires an informed agreement negotiated in partnership between the prescriber and the patient. That in turn means that the patient will need full and fair information and, as with any patient consent to treatment, it must be in a form that they can understand. Plainly, for patients with learning difficulties or communication problems this will mean extra effort and, perhaps, additional resource input, but the patient is entitled to expect that healthcare professionals will try to involve them in decisions about their treatment.

At the same time, the concordance approach places some responsibility on the patient too. They have had an opportunity to discuss their treatment and have made a voluntary commitment to taking it. This implies a more adult relationship than the old compliance approach.

Patient health: beliefs and concordance

To promote concordance the health professional must work with the patient to gain an understanding of the patient's health beliefs, the reasons for these, and the feelings, thoughts, and actions that these beliefs elicit in the patient (Aronson, 2007). This understanding of patient's health beliefs arguably supports achievement of a shared understanding, because you cannot reach any agreement if you do not know what the patient wants or hopes for from their treatment.

To engage the patient fully, we must incorporate the patient's perspective and monitor our own responses to that. This is an exercise in reflective practice and you may wish to use a framework to help you with

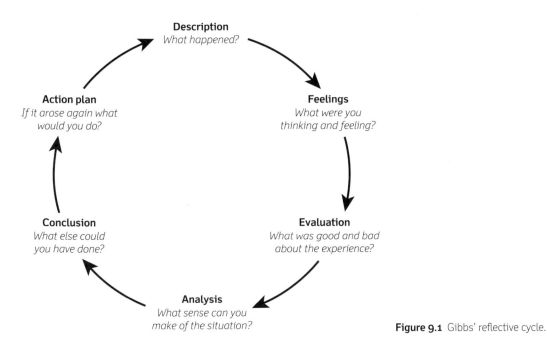

Figure 9.1 Gibbs' reflective cycle.

reflection. One example is Gibb's reflective cycle (1988) (Figure 9.1).

We must understand that our own health beliefs are only one set of many possibilities. Sometimes we do not realize that we even have 'health beliefs'—we think of them as facts—but if the patient's understanding of their health is different to our understanding, that will make it difficult to reach a genuine agreement.

For example, the patient may believe that all cancers are fatal, and if this is not corrected they may refuse treatment that could help them. They may think that pain is a necessary part of their condition, or that they 'deserve' it for some reason. However, we must be careful not to think that all patient beliefs need 'correcting'. Some are at least as valid as our own and all need to be taken into account.

To give them information, we must relate it to their understanding of their own health or illness. We need to provide opportunities for the patient to ask questions, seek clarification, or express doubts, and therefore we must have sufficient knowledge to be able to answer those questions or doubts or, if necessary, refer the patient to others who can. It is not enough to give the patient a chance to say their piece; we also have to listen to them. This seems obvious, but it is not

uncommon for patients to complain that though they repeatedly reported a problem, no action was taken because nobody seemed to be listening. We must also be aware of any non-verbal responses that communicate a patient's concerns. Our aim is to arrive jointly at an agreement that draws on the experiences, beliefs, and wishes of the patient to help them decide when, how, and why to use medicines.

Two factors which influence patient concordance are too often neglected. We must try to keep the regimen of drugs—that is, the types and frequencies of medicines taken—as simple as possible, because even a well-motivated patient will have difficulty keeping to an over-complicated plan. This might mean that we agree to a pattern that is not necessarily the best, but which is best for the patient in front of us. As an example, consider Stan. Stan is an 85-year-old man who takes tablets for his angina. Ideally we would like him to take them 12 hours apart, but when he took them at 7 am and 7 pm he frequently forgot the evening dose. However, his daughter usually called in or telephoned after work, so his evening dose was moved to 5 o'clock when his daughter could prompt him to take it. Stan and his doctor agreed that it was more important that he had two doses than that he stuck strictly to 12-hourly intervals.

A second problem is that patients frequently do not understand the reason for taking a medicine or what it is meant to achieve. The absence of a clear goal or strategy is a deterrent to the use of a drug. This is especially true when a drug is given prophylactically (to prevent a condition) rather than as a treatment. For example, if a patient has no symptoms, they need to be given a good reason to take a cholesterol-lowering drug for the rest of their lives.

Adherence

Once concordance has been reached, the patient chooses when and how to take their medicines based on the negotiation that they have had with the health professional. The term for this active choice in which the health professional and patient participate as equal partners is **adherence**.

Factors that promote adherence:

- Dependent on patient's lifestyle
- Ability to work with a regimen
- Consider side effects
- Patient choice
- Polypharmacy
- Dexterity
- Understanding.

Exercise 9.2

Can you think of other factors that might help to promote adherence? Make a list of them.

NICE (2009) have produced clinical guidelines on improving medicines adherence. This includes three key areas:

1 We must involve patients in decisions about medicines by:
Providing information
Increasing our understanding of the patient's perspective
Improving communication with patients
Increasing patient involvement in decision-making.

2 We must support adherence by:
Assessing adherence
Considering interventions to increase adherence.

3 We enhance adherence by:
Reviewing the medicines prescribed
Ensuring good communication between healthcare professionals.

The NICE guidelines can be viewed at: **http://guidance. nice.org.uk/CG76/Guidance/pdf/English**.

Concordance within the team

For medicines to be taken safely by the patient, it is important that concordance is achieved within the team; this means that health professionals must treat one another as partners and recognize each other's skills that can in turn be used to improve the patient's participation.

Reflection point

In light of this information, consider a recent consultation that you have had with a patient: What were the key components that made it successful?

Challenges to a concordant relationship

The ability to achieve a concordant relationship, that is, an agreement between the health professional, the patient, and/or the carer, is dependent on good two- or three-way communication. If there are barriers to communication, such as when working with patients who have visual, oral, or aural impairment, or who have mental impairment, then there might be difficulties in achieving a concordance. Take some time to think about this and consider the following scenario (Case study 9.1).

Concordance and consent

One way of viewing concordance is to consider it as a form of consent to medical treatment. Except in very limited circumstances, we would not operate surgically

Case study 9.1

Mrs Khan is a widow in her seventies. She came to the United Kingdom in her middle age and has never mastered English, but within her community this has not been a great disadvantage. Her son Masood speaks reasonable English but has a very traditional view of a man's place in the home. Since his father died, he has made all the big decisions for his mother. His daughter Fatima is 13 and speaks excellent English, but is not fluent in Urdu. Mrs Khan is also very deaf. Mrs Khan has developed diabetes and needs to take a metformin tablet with breakfast and tea and vary her diet. What difficulties could you foresee in helping her to do this?

Obviously there may be a language difficulty if you do not speak Urdu and Mrs Khan does not speak English. You might be able to communicate through her son or granddaughter, but remember that there may be confidentiality issues, and for this reason it is recommended that family translators are not used. Fatima may also be too young to help her grandmother and may not understand what is needed of her. It is possible that Masood believes that as the senior man of the family he is entitled to be involved in any discussions about his mother's care, and will not understand why you cannot agree to that. Without understanding the composition of a Pakistani diet it may be difficult for you to suggest dietary changes. Mrs Khan may also need counselling if she plans to fast during Ramadan. Even if you overcome these problems, you have to find a way of discussing your plans with a very deaf lady.

on a patient without clear consent, usually written, but we have not been in the habit of expecting the same process in the case of medical treatment. Yet those patients are just as entitled to that respect for their autonomy, and agreeing a course of drug treatment with them is no less important. Moreover, thinking of concordance as a type of consent should automatically bring the right considerations to our minds.

You may recall that for a person to be able to give a valid consent he or she must understand the information that they have been given; they must believe it to be true (or at least not disbelieve it); they must be capable of retaining all the information they need for as long as it takes them to make a decision; and they must be able to weigh information so as to make that decision. The decision they make may surprise us, but we cannot disregard it just because it is not the decision we have made. After all, people of full mental capacity make strange decisions all the time—you can see that from the clothes some of our friends buy or the football teams they choose to support.

The requirement to understand the information immediately suggests some of the allowances we may have to make. We may need to have material translated, or available in picture form, or offered in sign language for the deaf. Even if a patient can read English well, we must ensure that the leaflets we give them are written at a level that they can understand.

Achievement of a concordant relationship is also dependent on the patient's capacity to process information and to make a decision on the basis of their understanding of what has been said. This is often the case with patients who have certain forms of learning disability, damage to the brain, or other impairments that inhibit their ability to process information. However it would be wrong to assume that because a patient lacks the ability to process information on one level that it would not be possible to reach a mutual understanding between the patient and the health professional and that a concordant agreement on taking medicines cannot be achieved.

Adverse drug reactions and concordance

Adverse drug reactions and adherence are closely allied. Adherence is based on what is known as concordance, that is, a participative partnership agreement between the patient and the prescriber as to the medicine that they will take (Medicines Partnership, 2003). The term adherence is used to define what might happen as a result of a concordance being reached, that is, in an ideal world the patient will take their medicine as directed. Adherence by the patient to their medication regime is known to decline as increasing

Table 9.1 Defining concordance, adherence, and compliance, NICE (2009).

Concordance	A partnership agreement between the patient/carer, the nurse who is caring for the patient, and the prescriber based on an understanding of how, when, why, where, and how often to take medicine. For concordance to happen, the prescriber must first gain fully informed consent from the patient. The patient must be informed of potential effects and side effects and what to do if these occur.
Adherence	Taking medicine as agreed. Nurses can support patients in their care to do so and must themselves have an understanding of the medicine, its effects, and potential side effects and interactions.
Compliance	A term that is generally no longer used in relation to medicines management and which infers that the patient is following the instructions of the prescriber and or nurse who is caring for them without questioning and in spite of side effects and potential adverse reactions.

numbers of drugs are prescribed (Col et al, 1990). This may be overcome by improving communication within a good professional relationship between the prescriber, the professional who is managing the patient on a daily basis, and the patient (Rycroft-Malone, 2002). Reduced concordance may also arise because the patient's capacity to understand and retain information is impaired. However, there is also good evidence of intentional non-compliance, where patients deliberately chose to either disagree with the prescriber in the first instance, or deliberately chose not to adhere to their medication regime (Lowe and Raynor, 2000). Patients are encouraged to make choices based on the information that they have received, but if this is inaccurate or incomplete a lack of adherence to therapy may result (Westbury et al, 2003, Berry et al, 2000). The patient may stop taking the medicine if, for example, side effects are experienced which have not been explained (Ekman et al, 2007).

Conditions associated with patient ageing also introduce barriers to concordance. Dysphagia means the patient may be unable to swallow the medicine. Dysphagia is particularly a problem for patients who have conditions such as stroke or Parkinson's disease. One primary care survey found 11% of patients had difficulty in swallowing (Preston and Morris, 2005). Nurses may be able to suggest that prescribers could consider alternative formulations such as dispersible tablets or liquids, but you should seek pharmaceutical advice before suggesting tablet crushing as some tablets cannot be crushed without affecting their pharmacokinetics and their effects on the patient (Griffith, 2010). However, crumbling chewable tablets such as

calcium supplements immediately before administration may help patients to overcome chewing difficulties.

Other conditions such as arthritis may make it difficult for the patient to remove doses from the packaging and patients might be given devices to support them to open bottles and packets. These include special bottle caps such as winged caps (which have large flat surfaces like ears that the user can push to rotate the cap), or caps which can be opened by inserting a tool like a spanner into a hole. Alternatively the patient may request that child-resistant caps are not used. The Poppit™ device looks like a stapler and pushes a tablet out of a blister when it is placed on the base and the handle is pressed.

For some patients a monitored dosage system (MDS) (see Figure 9.2) may be appropriate. The dispenser removes the tablets or capsules from the manufacturers' packaging and seals them in a pack, usually 1 week in each pack. There are a number of different types of MDS.

In practice, the labels for the various medications would be attached to the front of the pack, but have been removed here to preserve patient confidentiality.

Patients posing particular difficulty

These may include people with learning difficulties, dementia, sensory impairment, or language difficulties. See also Chapter 5 for further discussion on groups at special risk.

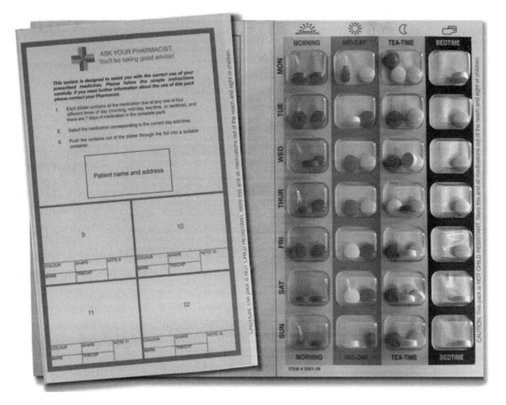

Figure 9.2 A monitored dosage system (or compliance pack).

Reflection point

Reflect on your experiences of supporting patients with difficulties.
What factors did you need to consider?

A range of difficulties can arise when attempting to promote concordance with any patients, but the potential increases when patients have particular difficulties. You will need to make a thorough assessment of the individual's needs.

You may have thought about the following issues:

- Understanding of the spoken word (some people may require an interpreter and written information in their own language about their medicines. Similarly, deaf or hard of hearing patients may need written information. Some people with learning difficulties may not be able to understand what you mean).
- Vision (you will need to think about how this patient will manage their medicines when they are discharged).

- Ability to read written material.
- Dexterity and coordination (this will need to be considered in advance of the patient being discharged).
- Is this individual able to consent? (see Chapter 1).

Learning disabilities or difficulties

It must be remembered that there are various levels of learning disability, which will need to be identified in order to include and ensure safety of the individual in the management of their medicines. Many are able to communicate using spoken language and, given the chance, can manage well (British Institute of Learning Disabilities, 2009). However, those with more profound difficulties will require more support and may have an advocate to ensure the individual's voice is heard. More information about advocacy is available at: **http://www/ bild.org.uk/information/factsheets/?locale=en**

Patients with dementia

Approximately 700 000 people in the UK have dementia (DH, 2009) so you are likely to be caring for patients with this condition at some time. People with dementia will often have limited cognitive resources by which to process information correctly, placing them at high risk of medication misadventure (Kralik et al, 2008). This may well be more of a problem when individuals are managing medicines within their own home.

Whilst in a care setting patients with dementia can be supervised in taking medicines appropriately and there are many ways to enable safe and effective medicine administration. One of the most widely used approaches for people with dementia is 'Reality Orientation' (Adams, 2008) and relies on staff providing the person with current information at every interaction with them. Maintaining genuine eye contact and using a clear but gentle voice can be reassuring for a person with dementia and can aid the building of trust, this is important when administering medicines.

Similarly, Kitwood (1997) suggests an approach towards people with dementia that involves collaboration. The idea is that the carer's words and actions should allow the person with dementia to feel they have done something themselves rather than having something done to them. Engaging in this way ensures the individual is given a sense of dignity and being valued.

Clearly, keeping people with dementia safe is vital and to do so you must be aware of potential dangers for the individual. This will need to be considered again if the patient is returning to their own home. Opportunities should be explored to provide information or training for carers on handling, administering, and storing medication for patients with dementia to increase safety and help to improve health and wellbeing outcomes (Royal Pharmaceutical Society, 2006).

Patients with impairment of vision

Some patients may be unable to read the written information provided with their medication. Since 2005 drug packaging must have the identity and strength of the contents displayed in Braille. The requirements can be found at **http://www.**

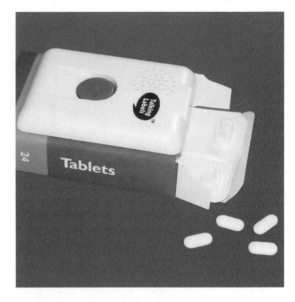

Figure 9.3 A Talking Label™.
Courtesy of Talking Products Ltd.

mhra.gov.uk/Howweregulate/Medicines/Label spatientinformationleafletsandpackaging/ Brailleonlabellingandinpatientinformationleaflets/ index.htm.

Some pharmacies are able to produce Braille labels for dispensed medicines. However, a better approach may be to attach pre-printed commercial Braille labels, because most pharmacists would not be able to read the label that they were attaching and would therefore not notice a mistake. Almost all pharmacies can produce large print labels for the poorly-sighted. An alternative is the talking label, a small voice-recording chip embedded in an adhesive plastic holder (see Figure 9.3). The pharmacist records the directions for use on the chip which can then be played by the patient by pressing the central button.

Preparing a patient for discharge

The administration of any medicine can be associated with the risk of an adverse event, side effect, or interaction, and it must be acknowledged that this risk may be increased when patients transfer from one setting to another—from home to hospital, from one hospital ward to another, or from hospital to intermediate care, a care home, or to their own home (The Royal Pharmaceutical Society, 2006).

As well as discussing medicines commenced while an in-patient, it is important to confirm that the patient understands how to correctly take any medicines which they were taking prior to admission. It is common to come across patients taking their oral iron preparations with a cup of tea, although they comment that they do vaguely remember being told that this is not advisable. Do not assume that if a patient has been on medication for some time that they are necessarily taking it appropriately: check this with them.

Preparing patients for discharge should start as soon as they are admitted (Gates, 2006) with particular attention to their medication needs.

You may have included some of the following factors:

Reflection point

Reflect on the issues regarding medicines management you need to consider when preparing patients for discharge.

- The number of medicines the patient will need.
- The patient's understanding of these medicines; how they work and how to take them.
- Is the patient clear about how long to continue medication? Do they know how to obtain further prescriptions?
- Can the patient manage to administer their medicines?
- If a carer needs to be involved do they have the understanding and ability to administer the medicines?
- Are there any special storage issues and can this be managed in the patient's home?

Various tools are available to help identify patients who may have difficulties in managing medicines if discharged home. Have a look at the following websites for further details: **http://www.pcc.nhs.uk/98.php** and **http://www.psnc.org.uk/publications_detail.php/94/moving_patient_moving_medicines_moving_safely_discharge_and_transfer_planning**.

It is important always to check that the patient understands how and when to take their medicines

before they are discharged from hospital. The patient should be given written information on how to do this and also the patient's community doctor (GP) must be provided with the same information for the patient notes. It is also important that the GP is able to access discharge information quickly, and many areas are now developing fast, effective ways of communicating confidential information between hospital and community care.

Can you think of good practice when communicating between professionals in the areas in which you have worked?

If you are involved in this process remember to check that the patient understands which medicines to take and also remember to check whether they have other medicines at home that they might start to take without agreement. Make it clear to the patient that they should only take the medicines that have been prescribed for them on discharge and if in doubt make sure that you advise their community nurse/GP.

Planning for an effective discharge takes time. It should not be left until the transport is on its way to collect your patient. Remember that most of us can only assimilate a certain amount of new information in one sitting, so if you have a lot of new messages, consider how you can spread them over a day or two.

When discussing patients' medicines at any stage it is important to acknowledge that some patients will have become experts in the management of their own medicines. Always find out what the patient already knows and understands.

Expert patient programme

By working towards achieving concordance with patients we encourage them to participate in decision making. With information about their medical condition and its treatment the outcome, over time, can often result in individuals with expert knowledge.

With many more people living beyond their 70s and 80s, there are increasing numbers of people living with long-term conditions, such as heart disease, diabetes, and arthritis. Overall, 15.4 million people, or almost one in three of the population, in England has a long-term condition (DH, 2008) and many become 'experts'.

Reflection point

> Reflect on your experiences of patients who were 'experts' about their medical condition.
>
> Do you always try and find out what patients know about their condition?
>
> Consider how you feel when patients know more than you. Does this affect the way in which you interact with them?

Expert patients:

- Feel confident and in control of their lives
- Aim to manage their condition and its treatment in partnership with health care professionals
- Communicate effectively with professionals and are willing to share responsibility and treatment
- Are realistic about the impact of their disease on themselves and their family
- Use their skills and knowledge to lead full lives.

(DH, 2007)

The benefits of encouraging patients to become experts in their medical condition include achieving improved health outcomes and reducing use of healthcare services (DH, 2007). A literature review (Barlow et al, 2002) identified the following benefits for patients when they were able to self-manage their condition:

- Reduced severity of symptoms
- Significant decrease in pain
- Improved life control and activity
- Improved resourcefulness and life satisfaction.

The Expert Patients Programme aims to support people living with long-term conditions. It is a lay-led self-management programme that has been specifically developed to increase patients' confidence, improve their quality of life, and enable them to better manage their condition (DH, 2007).

Summary

This chapter explored the theory of concordance and has provided a range of information to enable you to understand the concept. It has also detailed some of the circumstances you might need to consider when working in partnership with patients to achieve concordance, thus ensuring individuals make safe and appropriate decisions that suit their needs.

References

Adams T (2008), *Dementia Care Nursing*. Basingstoke: Palgrave Macmillan.

Aronson J (2007). Compliance, concordance, adherence, *British Journal of Clinical Pharmacology*, 63; 383–384.

Barlow J, Wright C, Sheasby J, Turner A, and Hainsworth J (2002). Self-management approaches for people with chronic conditions: a review, *Patient Education and Counseling*, 48; 177–187.

Berry CA, Bradley CP, Brittain N, Stevenson FA, and Barber N (2000). Patients' unvoiced agenda in general practice consultations: qualitative study, *BMJ*, 320; 1246–1250.

British Institute of Learning Disabilities (BILD) (2009) Fact Sheets. Available at: http://www.bild.org.uk/information/factsheets/?locale=en (accessed on 4 March 2012).

Col N, Fanale JE, and Kronholm P (1990). The role of medication noncompliance and adverse drug reactions in hospitalizations of the elderly, *Archives of Internal Medicine*, 150; 841–845.

Department of Health (2007), The Expert Patients' Programme. Available at: http://www.dh.gov.uk/en/Aboutus/MinistersandDepartmentLeaders/ChiefMedicalOfficer/ProgressOnPolicy/ProgressBrowsableDocument/DH_5380856 (accessed on 17 September 2009).

Department of Health (2008), Ten things you need to know about long term conditions. Available at: http://www.dh.gov.uk/en/Healthcare/Longtermconditions/DH_084294 (accessed on 17 September 2009).

Department of Health (2009) Living Well With Dementia: A National Dementia Strategy. Available at: http://www.dh.gov.uk/prod_consum_dh/groups/dh_digitalassets/documents/digitalasset/dh_103136.pdf (accessed on 25 September 2009).

Ekman I, Schaufelberger M, Kjellgren KI, Swedberg K. and Granger BB (2007). Standard medication information is not enough: poor concordance of patient and nurse perceptions, *Journal of Advanced Nursing*, 60; 181–186.

Gates C (2006). Drug history taking—avoiding the common pitfalls, *Hospital Pharmacist*, 13; 98–100.

Gibbs G (1988) *Learning by Doing: A guide to teaching and learning methods*. Oxford: Further Education Unit, Oxford Polytechnic.

Griffith R (2010). Managing medication Compliance. *British Journal of Healthcare Management*, 16; 402–408.

Kitwood T (1997), *Dementia Reconsidered*. Buckingham: Open University Press.

Kralik D, Visentin K, March G, Anderson B, Gilbert A, and Boyce M (2008). Medication Management for Community-dwelling Older People with Dementia and Chronic Illness, *Australian Journal of Primary Care*, 14; 25–35.

Lowe CJ and Raynor DK (2000). Intentional nonadherence in elderly patients: fact or fiction? *Pharmaceutical Journal* 265: 19.

Medicines Partnership (2003), Project evaluation toolkit, in Courtenay M, and Griffiths M (2010), *Independent and Supplementary Prescribing: An essential guide*. Cambridge: Cambridge University Press, p 112.

National Institute for Health and Clinical Excellence (2009), Medicines Adherence. Involving patients in decisions about prescribed medicines and supporting adherence: http://www.nice.org.uk/nice-media/pdf/CG76NICEGuideline.pdf (accessed 10 May 2012).

The Nursing and Midwifery Council (2008), *The code: Standards of conduct, performance and ethics for nurses and midwives*. London: NMC.

Osterberg L, and Blaschke T (2005). Drug therapy: Adherence to Medication, *New England Journal of Medicine*, 353; 487–497.

Preston M, and Morris H (2005). Medication and dysphagia, *General Practitioner*, 11 February, p 62.

The Royal Pharmaceutical Society of Great Britain (RPSGB), The Guild of Hospital Pharmacists, The Pharmaceutical Services Negotiating Committee, and The Primary Care Pharmacists' Association (2006) *Moving patients, Moving Medicines, Moving Safely:Guidance on Discharge and Transfer Planning*. Available at: http://www.psnc.org.uk/publications_detail.php/94/moving_patient_moving_medicines_moving_safely_discharge_and_transfer_planning (accessed on 15 June 2012).

Rycroft-Malone J (2002), Patient Participation in Nurse-patient Interactions About Medication (unpublished PhD thesis, School of Nursing and Midwifery, University of Southampton) in Courtenay M, and Griffiths M (2005), *Independent and Supplementary Prescribing: An essential guide*, Cambridge: Cambridge University Press, pp. 121–33.

Westbury J, Pollock K, and Blenkinsopp A (2003). A study of concordance issues in older people, *The International Journal of Pharmacy Practice*, 11 [Supplement].

World Health Organization (2003), *Adherence to Long-Term Therapies: Evidence for Action*. Geneva: World Health Organization.

10 Keeping Up to Date

CHAPTER CONTENTS

- Introduction
- New roles and organizations
- Medicines and change management
- Working with others
- Clinical governance and patient safety
- Clinical audit
- Risk management

- Workforce issues
- Clinical supervision
- Competencies and revalidation
- Delegation
- Specialized skills for particular settings
- Summary

LEARNING OUTCOMES

- To gain an understanding of strategies that can be used to keep your skills in medicines management up to date, including clinical supervision and change management.
- To acknowledge the implications of clinical governance as related to keeping up to date within medicines management.

Introduction

It is hoped that this book will provide a useful resource in the future to help keep your skills and knowledge up to date. This final chapter covers some of the strategies that may help. It will discuss some of the relevant developments and offer some thoughts about future advances in medicines management.

The world of medicines management is constantly evolving although, having said that there are given constants and principles that will remain the same in all settings. For example, patient safety is obviously in the forefront of all practice as is efficacy of treatment and effective resource management.

As explained within the context of this book there are a number of ways of ensuring that the instructions for giving medicines are clear and that medicines are legally and safely dispensed, supplied, and administered to patients. Other terms for ways to dispense, supply, or administer medicines are **process** or **mechanism**.

Exercise 10.1

Can you remember the different legal mechanisms for the dispensing, supply, and administration of medicines? See Chapter 1 to check on your answers.

Some of these mechanisms have been in place for many years; for example, before the Medicines Act 1968. Others have been enforced more recently; non-medical prescribing only came into being in the mid-1990s and continues to expand in the current decade (Association for Nurse Prescribers). It can be safely stated that all of the legal mechanisms for the dispensing, supply, and administration of medicines have been reviewed and tightened up either locally, nationally, or both within the last 10 years. This reinforcement has occurred because of the following factors; you may be able to think of more:

- Concerns about patient safety and medicines management.
- Directives for a changing and evolving health service moving, for example, towards the management of the care of patients with long term conditions in the community setting.
- Delivery of medicines management by more advanced non-medical healthcare practitioners other than doctors, such as nurses and pharmacists.
- As a result of the Fourth Shipman Report. (2004).

Non-medical prescribing by advanced nurses and other designated health practitioners has challenged pre-existing practice and supported the enforcement of local and national policies for the safe and effective management of medicines. The mechanism of non-medical prescribing can be shown to save time and to effectively manage the patient's condition and has been proven to be both effective and cost effective (Latter et al, 2005). For example before community nurses were able to train as non-medical prescribers they would often have to wait outside the doctor's office to acquire a prescription. In the same way non-medical prescribers within a hospital setting can now write up prescriptions on the patient's medical administration record (MAR) rather than wait for a junior doctor to do so. The advantage to the patient is not limited to giving better access to treatment. It is arguable that an experienced nurse who has worked in a particular area of practice for some time may be more familiar with the medicines used than a junior doctor whose experience has previously been elsewhere.

Other mechanisms such as patient specific directions and patient group directions (see Chapter 1) for the dispensing, supply, and administration of drugs are still in place, and are useful. Providing they are used appropriately, they are effective tools for getting the correct medicine to the correct patient in a timely and safety-conscious fashion. It is of course important that when you are dealing with medicines and patients you are aware of the mechanism for supply or administration that is being used and that you adhere to local and national policy (DH, 2006a and NMC 2008a).

In the last decade, healthcare delivery was focused on transferring care for patients with long term conditions from the acute setting into the community. There was an emphasis on delivering care to the patient by those healthcare professionals who were best-placed to do this effectively, with the capability to review and amend care accordingly. There has been greater focus on the prevention of acute exacerbation of long term conditions such as diabetes, coronary heart disease, and Parkinson's disease, and although further research still needs to be done, the role of the advanced healthcare practitioner as a non-medical prescriber has been particularly beneficial. Services have been encouraged to enable patients to access care in an appropriate setting and in a timely fashion, and for that care to be carried out by the professional who is best equipped to do so. For example, walk-in centres that are staffed by registered healthcare practitioners who are competent to follow the directions in a PGD but who are not doctors have, and are likely to, continue to meet this remit into the future.

The great advantages of PGDs are that they allow patients quick access to medicines and can be operated by a range of suitably trained practitioners, greatly increasing the number of settings in which supply can be made. As noted in Chapter 1, non-medical prescribing retains clear accountability of a particular professional to the patient and allows the professional a wider range of treatment options. It may therefore be desirable for non-medical prescribing to grow and for PGDs to be used less as a result. However, the MHRA (2010) have some concerns that PGDs are being used to 'cope with shortages of staff with prescribing qualifications . . . and may be an obstacle to non-medical prescribers attaining independent prescribing qualifications'. There are also concerns they are being increasingly used to 'manage planned care, as distinct from unannounced clinical need, and no longer meet the original intention that they should be reserved for those limited situations where this offers a distinct advantage for patient care.'

You may, at this stage, want to consider the use of PGDs within your area of practice versus independent non-medical prescribers.

It is likely that the delivery of healthcare will continue to evolve and that greater responsibilities for care of patients will be further moved into both the community and independent sector. With a greater emphasis on training within the pre-registration curriculum on medicines management and with the need for advanced specialist practitioners to have a prescribing qualification it means that nurses and other registered health professionals might well be able to deliver a truly holistic service both initiating and completing the package of care. Although challenging, with an emphasis on professional accountability, patient satisfaction, cost consciousness, and safety, it is arguably an exciting time to be a healthcare professional.

Prescribing can be seen as a logical extension of the nursing role and with pre-registration programmes including more pharmacology it may be a natural progression for nurses, in the future, to become prescribers at an earlier stage than currently.

The non-medical prescribing programme has already proved very popular with nurses. In July 2010 over 40000 nurses were practising as non-medical prescribers in primary care, 11000 of these as independent/supplementary prescribers (NHSBSA, 2010). Numbers for secondary care are unknown, but would have to be added to these to give a complete picture.

New roles and organizations

We live and work within a constantly changing environment. As such, it is difficult to predict the changes that will occur for you when you gain registration and throughout your professional journey. However, the one predictable thing is that change will happen.

You might find that in your professional lifetime you work for many different employing organizations. It is probable that not all of these will come under the auspices of what has, until now, been recognized as the National Health Service. For example, doctors and pharmacists now consult in supermarkets and there are walk-in centres in station forecourts. Regardless of where you work and by whom you are employed, you need to be very clear that you have read and understood your employer's medicines policy and any other directions pertaining to the supply and administration of medicines, and that you are working within your

professional code of conduct, performance, and ethics (NMC, 2008b), and to the standards for medicines management and any further guidance regarding the supply and administration of medicines that might come from the NMC who are your professional body (NMC, 2010a).

Medicines and change management

The past 10 years have seen great changes in the role of the nurse with increasing responsibilities and an increased awareness of accountability, not least in the area of medication management. There have also been huge organizational changes. Change can be very unsettling, particularly for nurses who as health professionals need to feel that they can predict and manage outcome for their patients. Trying to navigate our way through all of the changes can be likened to navigating a sailing boat in a storm. You need a triangulation point on which to focus and although you cannot always head in a straight line towards it, you have something to aim for. In the case of medicines management, our navigation points are our policies and procedures, based on the principles of best evidence and of clinical governance. The point is that different organizations will have different policies and protocols under which you will be given responsibilities. It is important that, whichever organization you work for, you are aware of these.

All employing healthcare organizations will be required to meet a set of minimum standards regarding medicines management and these, as previously noted in this book, are set down by the Department of Health and the Care Quality Commission (DH, 2006b). These standards are the national minimum benchmarks to which all organizations who are dealing with the management of medicines must adhere and so it is important that you are aware of them. These are **minimum** standards: best practice may place higher requirements on us. They are also fixed, whereas our developing practice should enable us to see opportunities to improve upon them. Your main point of navigation is, as a nurse, the NMC *Standards for Medicines Management* (NMC, 2010a); more can be found regarding this in

Chapter 1, including details of the *Essential skills cluster: Medicines management* (NMC, 2010b).

When considering our own reaction to change we should, as professionals, use reflective practice to examine our own beliefs, values, attitudes, and assumptions and continually challenge these. In so doing, we will be better placed to interact with our employing organization when change is suggested and to put the changes into the context of national and local drivers.

There are several theories as to what makes change happen. Davidhizar (1996) enquired about changes in healthcare in the 1990s and suggested that the factors that contributed to the changes in the system were as follows:

- Technology
- Information availability
- Growing populations.

Although the 1990s seem a long time ago, these factors are still relevant today.

Another major change has been in the skill mix of staff. Change in the work force has partly arisen due to shortage of doctors and a decrease in junior doctors' hours. Practices such as non-medical prescribing, and new standards for medicines management (NMC, 2010a and the *Essential Skills Cluster: Medicines Management* (NMC, 2010b) have happened partly out of necessity, in order to meet the demands of an increasingly elderly population who are living longer and because of a shortage of doctors to care for them.

Reflection point

Have you observed any other factors that have influenced change in your own work experience? You may like to list them and consider what effect these had on individuals.

It can be difficult for individuals to change and it is not uncommon to feel threatened, stressed, and bereft by the pace of events (Marquis and Houston, 2000). Lewin (1951) was the first to identify a theory of change and coin the term 'change agent'. His theories are still of significance today. A change agent is instrumental in leading and creating change within a system and in encouraging, inspiring, and supporting others to change. Lewin identified the process of change as being made up of three parts as follows:

- **Unfreezing:** where the change agent persuades others who are resistant to change that there is a valid reason to change.
- **Movement:** where there needs to be a balance between the need to change and the resistance to changing. The movement towards change should be gradual, where possible, with those who are resistant being supported and encouraged by the change agent towards new ways of doing things.
- **Refreezing:** where the change agent supports others to adapt to and to adopt and assimilate change into their normal working lives.

Sibler (1993) suggested that ability to change depends on an individual's approach to life events and their flexibility. Your own ability to adapt to change will be dependent on your personality, and the life experiences that you have already had to tackle. Ability to deal with change also rests on group and individual assessment of the impact of the changes on themselves and on others and on the perceived positive or negative outcomes of that change. It is likely that within a group of people undergoing change, there will be as many different ways of viewing the situation as there are members of the group.

Reflection point

Pause for a moment to consider the changes that you have already experienced in your life as a student and of the impact on yourself, your organization, and your colleagues. Now complete the following reflective exercise.

- What was the catalyst for the change (why did it happen and what made it happen)?
- Was there a change agent and who were they?
- How flexible have you been in relation to the change?
- How do you think you have adapted to the change?
- What has been the outcome (perceived and actual) for you personally and for the organization?
- How would you do things differently next time?
- And what have you learned as a result?

Working with others

The government agenda is that the patient has convenient access to the professional who is best able to treat their condition in the timeliest fashion (DH, 2009). You will have noticed that in your clinical practice nurses are not the only professionals who are involved in the administration of medicines or in prescribing. In addition to doctors and dentists and nurse prescribers, there are also pharmacist prescribers and growing numbers of allied health professionals, such as physiotherapists and podiatrist prescribers. With regards to the prescribing, dispensing, supply, and administration of medicines there can be overlap between the different professions and there is increasing blurring of the different professional boundaries and roles.

Picture one patient who has several different long-term conditions for example an older lady (Mrs X) who has diabetes and heart disease, who might also suffer from chronic obstructive pulmonary disease and osteoarthritis. How many professionals might she see in a six month period if her conditions remain stable? It is likely that she will see her GP who makes her initial diagnoses, the practice nurse who might administer her flu jab and dress her leg ulcer, the podiatrist who might treat an infected toe nail, the pharmacist who issues her with repeat prescriptions and the physiotherapist for mobility purposes. Now if any of these conditions worsen and lead to an acute exacerbation the number of professionals that she sees might double. Each of the professionals mentioned here has the ability to become a prescriber and each can administer medicines and some are able to dispense and supply. This may result in polypharmacy, the risks of which were described in Chapter 5. It is therefore of utmost importance that all the people who are involved in the care of Mrs X communicate clearly with each other.

Mrs X's GP is central to her care when she is stable and living at home. The GP is responsible for making the diagnoses of Mrs X's conditions and will refer to other professionals for more specialist care to be provided where necessary. A copy of Mrs X's medical notes will be held on computer by the GP and these are known as the central electronic record. When dealing with medicines, good record keeping and communication between professionals is fundamental to patient safety. Any prescribing decision, for example any change of medication or of dose, should be uploaded contemporaneously (straight away) into Mrs X's central electronic records. This might be difficult if for example the district nurse is dealing with Mrs X's diabetic insulin requirements on a Friday evening when the surgery is shut. However, best practice is that the records should be amended within 48 hours (with allowance to cover bank holidays), as recommended by the NMC (2006, p 28). The NMC (2009) *Guidance on Record Keeping for Nurses and Midwives* (p 1) states that:

> **Good record keeping is an integral part of nursing and midwifery practice, and is essential to the provision of safe and effective care. It is not an optional extra to be fitted in if circumstances allow.**

Clinical governance and patient safety

Clinical governance is defined as:

> **A system through which National Health Services (NHS) organizations are accountable for continuously improving the quality of their services and safeguarding high standards of care by creating an environment in which excellence in clinical care will flourish.**
>
> Scally and Donaldson, 1998, p 62.

In essence it is about learning from our mistakes and using that learning to inform an implement a high quality service. The culture within organizations should be one that sees errors and failings as spurs for improvement rather than as reasons for blame.

As nurses we must know when we have sufficient knowledge and skills (competence) to enable us to practise safely. We must also acknowledge the limitations of our competency and must not practice outside of the scope of our practice or outside of our own level of competence (NMC, 2008b).

In the past two decades there have been several high profile incidents that have alerted the medical and nursing world and the Department of Health to the fact that not enough was being done to ensure that we as professionals were practising safely and that our patients were being protected.

Clinical governance was central to a Department of Health White Paper (DH, 1998) and remains important today. The Care Quality Commission (CQC) state that it is important for providers of healthcare to have a strong system of clinical governance in place. The CQC (2010) provides guidance to ensure that the requirements of the Health and Social Care Act 2008 (Regulated Activities) Regulations 2010 and the Care Quality Commission (Registration) Regulations 2009 are met by care providers. Outcome 9 of this publication relates specifically to management of medicines.

There will be different ways in which the organization you work within ensures it meets the requirements of clinical governance. The Royal College of Nursing (2012) website includes information to ensure you keep up to date with clinical governance matters. In the next section a two examples of activities used for meeting clinical governance requirements will be discussed and related to the management of medicines. These are clinical audit and risk management.

Clinical audit

You might well have observed that practitioners are involved in several different types of clinical audit. Audit involves the collecting and bringing together (collating) of simple information and then examining this against professional standards, national and organizational policies and protocols to:

● Ensure that the above are being met

● Highlight and applaud good practice

● Make recommendations as to where and how practice might be improved.

Audited data are compared with similar data from different clinical areas or across clinical boundaries. Audit should be integral to practice and ongoing in the form of a cycle (see Figure 10.1). For example once the need to improve in an area has been identified, this is

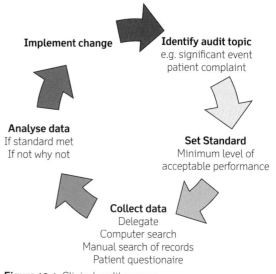

Figure 10.1 Clinical audit process.

fed back into the audit cycle and the improvements are monitored and reported on.

A common form of audit in the medicines management arena is the collection of prescribing data. In community practice, this is usually provided by ePACT data. The name comes from an earlier paper-based system called PACT (prescribing analysis and cost tool), which has been superseded by an online alternative.

ePACT allows the pharmaceutical and prescribing advisors of a primary care trust to analyse the previous 60 months' prescribing data. These data are updated on a monthly basis and can be selected according to prescriber, practice, drug, formulation, or month. Advisors then create reports for prescribers that allow them to see what they have been prescribing and compare them with others.

Such data have to be interpreted, but they can be illuminating. For example, if you find that someone is prescribing more antibiotics than a colleague in the same area of practice, are they prescribing too much, or is their colleague prescribing too little? Sometimes they will show that we choose more expensive medicines than our fellow prescribers, or give larger quantities.

If you know a nurse prescriber you could ask if they would be willing to show you the information that they receive. ePACT does not record any patient details, and these are normally concealed for hospital systems too. Prescribing advisors do not need or want patient information, because their interest is in patterns of prescribing rather than individual prescriptions.

If patient information is needed, advisors would normally ask the prescriber to review their records to collate it, but would expect patient data to be anonymized before it is sent in. For example, if a Trust discovers that a nurse prescriber who works in a diabetes clinic has been prescribing sleeping tablets, it may ask the nurse to justify this. It will not be able to identify the patients concerned, but by giving a date when the prescription was dispensed it may be possible for the nurse to find the details from her records. There may be a good reason that justifies the prescribing, or it may be poor practice.

Sometimes Trusts want to audit practice in a particular area of work. In a recent audit conducted by one of the authors, his Trust was concerned that strong analgesic medicines (fentanyl and tramadol) were being prescribed by professionals (both doctors and nurses) who appeared not to have been trained to use them. By reviewing the notes it was possible to discover that these were usually being prescribed to continue treatment when the patient had run out of stock. The prescribers felt obliged to prescribe outside their area of practice rather than let the patient go without; a better solution would be to ensure that patients' needs are reviewed earlier by properly trained colleagues.

Students and new registrants are unlikely to be involved in prescribing audits, but there will also be audits relating to administration of medicines. For example, on hospital wards, pharmacy staff will review notes to check that the administration records are being properly signed, that medicines are only being issued by people who have been trained to do so, and that best practice is being followed. A common audit is to check the administration times of medicines. In a large ward, it may not be practical to give all the medicines at precisely the best time, but by auditing the times it may become clear that practice is poor. For example, antibiotics that should be given half an hour before meals may be given too late; patients who should receive one tablet before meals and another after them may be given them simultaneously; and sometimes audit shows that sleeping tablets are used too often, or too early in the evening so patients wake during the night.

Reflection point

Reflect on your experiences of ensuring patients receive medicines at the correct time.

Noting that the CQC guidance states people 'will have their medicines at the times they need them, and in a safe way' (CQC, 2010, p104) consider how you might achieve this.

Risk management

To ensure the safe and effective management of medicines there is a need to recognize your responsibilities; one of these is to recognize the potential risks involved. Risk management is an important activity within clinical governance.

There have been several national, high profile cases involving the misuse of medicines and leading to the death of many patients. Among the most infamous is the case involving Beverly Allitt, a staff nurse on a paediatric unit, who induced insulin-related comas in the children on the unit by injecting them with insulin (Department of Health, 1994; The Times, 2007). Another case involved the general practitioner, Harold Shipman, who was deliberately causing the death of his patients by injecting them with diamorphine (Shipman Inquiry, 2005). Both the aforementioned individuals were registered professionals who abused the trust of the public by their actions. The inquiries into the incidents indicated that the amount of harm could have been reduced if certain processes had been in place within the organizations in which they worked. Whilst risk management can significantly diminish the harm that an individual is able to do to patients, we cannot entirely remove the risk of future harm by an individual who is determined to abuse their patients' trust. However, all employing organizations have a legal duty of care to their patients; part of this duty is to identify any loopholes within their systems and underpinning policies that might lead to a potential risk of the patient coming to harm.

The Department of Health (2006b) *Standards for Better Health*, recommended that all healthcare organizations, in both the private and public health sectors, who were acting as employers ensured that their staff worked to a set of minimum standards that included those for medicines management.

In addition all health organizations are required to have a medicines policy in place that will define the protocols and procedures for the safe administration of medicines, and individual nurses have a duty to work within the standards laid down by the NMC (2010a) *Standards for Medicines Management*.

We cannot consider risk management without some reference to workforce issues. You may have identified in the previous reflective exercise that factors related to the whole healthcare team impact on your ability to work in the ways that you strive for.

Workforce issues

James Reason (NPSA, 2008) described a theory of error causation which is known as Reason's three bucket model. His analogy pictures us carrying three buckets labelled self, context, and task. See Figure 10.2.

The **Self** bucket is the one that we all bring to work with us—the one that contains the car breaking down, the bank overdraft, and you feeling under the weather with a cold.

The **Context** bucket is when three other people who are on your shift with you are off sick with flu, your unit is closing because of MRSA, and your manager wants you to work unpaid overtime.

The **Task** bucket consists of the many different and competing demands on your clinical time during the course of a working day. For example, you are in the middle of helping Mrs X to take her medicines, when Mrs Y falls out of bed, and Dr Z wants you to help him to examine Mr G.

As nurses, we must carry all three buckets. How we manage all of these buckets in a professional way is not only dependent on our level of knowledge, skills, and competence, but also on what is going on in our personal lives. The contents of these buckets will be different for everybody. Reason's point is that you can probably manage to carry all three of these buckets without spilling anything, provided that they are not too full, or even when two of the buckets are nearly full. When any one of the buckets is so full that the water starts to slop over the edge, you could slip up; and when all three buckets are close to full at once, it is a disaster waiting to happen.

We all have an individual responsibility to highlight when our buckets are too full; and our managers have a responsibility to do something about those concerns through systematic review of our workload balance, and by identifying plans to address insufficiencies in resourcing. Although we cannot always predict whether our personal buckets are filling up, we have a duty to look after ourselves; this is often something that we as individuals are not so good at doing. We also have a duty to highlight our concerns about the poor practice of other professionals. This is not easy to do and the

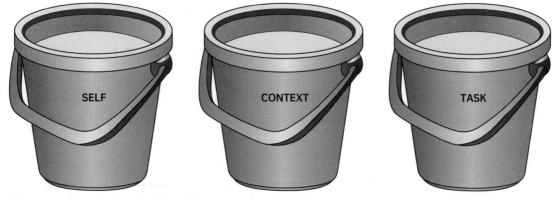

Figure 10.2 Reason's three bucket model.

NMC (2010c) has published guidance on raising and escalating concerns.

Healthcare professionals are sometimes too inclined to accept that there will always be errors, or that some things in their working lives cannot be changed. They may say, for example, that there is no point in complaining that their ward is understaffed because no spare staff will be available. However, if we believe that staffing numbers or quality are putting patients at risk, we have no ethical choice but to voice our concern—and to continue doing so. Maybe our employers can do little about the 'self' bucket, but if we think our performance is affected, we have a duty to let our line managers know.

As a nurse you have a duty of care to identify and minimize any potential risk (NMC, 2008b; NMC, 2010c) and this can be achieved in the following ways:

- Active clinical supervision
- Continuing professional development (CPD)
- Yellow card reporting and internal reporting of incidents/adverse drug reactions (see Chapter 2 for details).

Clinical supervision

It is an essential part of the NMC requirement for Prep (2006) that you seek regular professional supervision and build this into your time. As part of clinical governance, clinical supervision needs to be an on-going and regular occurrence throughout your professional lifetime. The purpose of supervision is to support patient safety by helping you to maintain standards, stay up to date, and work within your competence. Keep a record of your supervision and you will find that this will help you to prioritize the demands that are put on you.

The NMC have produced guidance regarding clinical supervision (NMC, 2008c). Basically they advise that clinical supervision is best when it takes place locally and addresses local need. The reasons that the NMC wish you to undertake supervision are to improve patient/client care by:

- Identifying solutions to problems
- Increasing the registrant's understanding of professional issues

- Further developing the registrant's skills and knowledge
- Enhancing their understanding of their own practice.

Ideally clinical supervision should be facilitated by a skilled supervisor who also has knowledge of your field and scope of practice. It can take several different forms and some suggestions for the way in which you might like to participate are set out here:

- Regular one-to-one sessions with an experienced supervisor
- Regular peer supervision on a one-to-one or group basis (facilitated by an experienced supervisor).

Exercise 10.2

There are other ways in which you can access supervision. Can you think of some?

Suggested topics that you might need to address in professional supervision are as follows:

- Matters that arise as part of your day-to-day work and that have caused you concern or that you wish to celebrate
- Workload issues (how full are your buckets)? (NPSA, 2008)
- Issues that have arisen as a result of changes to your practice
- Critical incidents that might have occurred and in which you might or might not have been involved.

Competencies and revalidation

You must keep your knowledge and skills up to date, using the best available evidence (NMC, 2008b) and this applies to all areas of your practice. It is therefore important for all registrants to ensure they keep up their competence in medicines management. Reference to the latest guidance from the NMC is vital. Equally, you must ensure that you always refer to the latest edition of sources such as the *BNF*.

Think for a moment about the resources that are available to you in your everyday practice and how you know where to look for guidance if, for example, you come across a medicine that you are unfamiliar with. You will find appropriate resources that may be useful in Chapter 6.

As previously stated nurses are required by the NMC to undertake and record their continuing professional development (NMC, 2008b). The Prep handbook (NMC, 2008b) gives clear guidance on the requirements, including the need to undertake at least 35 hours of learning activity relevant to your practice during a 3-year period. There are no approved learning activities but you could, for example, document your increasing knowledge and competence in medicine management, using reference to elements of this book. For example, your increased understanding of the pharmacokinetics and pharmacodynamics of a drug that you were less familiar with could be recorded and the implications for your practice highlighted.

There are mandatory CPD requirements for prescribers; in the case of nurses to ensure they are able to continue to meet the NMC *Standards of Proficiency for Nurse and Midwife Prescribers* (2006). In order to achieve this prescribers need access to evidence-based development opportunities. The NMC (2008c) also recommends that prescribers should have their 'prescribing' role appraised annually as part of their performance review.

Delegation

When you become a registered nurse, you will be able under certain circumstances to delegate the supply and administration of medicines to others with whom you work. You must be very clear about what you are able to delegate, to whom, and under what circumstances.

Who can delegate and to whom?

A **doctor** can write a prescription and can delegate the supply and/or administration of medicines to other registered health professionals.

A **registered nurse**, who holds the recordable qualification of Nurse Independent and Supplementary Prescriber, can delegate the administration of medicines that they have prescribed to another professional, a healthcare assistant, the carer, or to the patient. The nurse must firstly ensure that the person that they are delegating to is competent (has the knowledge and skills) to be able to safely supply or administer the medicine. The registered nurse is accountable for assessing the competence of the person to whom they delegate. The registered nurse must not delegate to a person that they do not deem to be competent.

A **registered nurse** who is not a prescriber can delegate the administration of medicines to a healthcare assistant, another registered nurse, the patient, or the carer providing that the medicines have in the first instance been prescribed by a doctor, dentist, or non-medical prescriber. In common speech we refer to the piece of paper on which a doctor orders a medicine as a prescription, but the prescription is the instruction, not the paper. The prescription can take the form of an FP10 (a standard NHS prescription in England), a medicines administration record, a private prescription, or it can be written in the patient's notes. All these will be for a particular patient, so generically they are known as patient specific directions or PSDs. The nurse must firstly ensure that the person to whom they delegate is competent (has the knowledge and skills) to be able to safely supply or administer the medicine. Again, it is the responsibility of the registered nurse to assess the competency of the person to whom they have delegated. The registered nurse must not delegate to a person who they do not deem to be competent.

Student nurses: the NMC (2008b) is very clear that students are not permitted to supply or administer medicines to a patient except under direct supervision. Direct supervision means that the supervisor is in a position to intervene immediately if necessary.

What cannot be delegated?

A registered nurse is not permitted to delegate the supply or administration of medicines to another person if they are working within the parameters of a patient group direction (see Chapter 7 for more information on the supply and administration of medicines). This is because the organization that is responsible for having written the PGD is already delegating to the registered professionals who are named on the PGD and it is not possible to sub-delegate. In addition the NMC is very clear that registered nurses who are named on the PGD are not allowed to delegate the supply or administration of medicines to a student nurses as this again would be sub-delegating. If you are a student nurse and are reading this and have been asked to administer or supply medicines that have been authorized by a PGD, please be very clear that you are not permitted to do so (NMC, 2008a). A PGD is an authority given to particular professionals named within it. That authority cannot be passed on to others who are not named.

Specialized skills for particular settings

Depending on the area of clinical practice you work in your knowledge and competence in medicines management will develop for the medicines you are using for the patients in your care. For example, those working with children will become familiar with the complexity of dosages. The *BNF for Children* was published to help practitioners working with children and should be used for paediatric medicine management. Nurses who prescribe for children should only do so if they have the relevant knowledge, experience, and competence in nursing children (NMC, 2006).

As you progress through your healthcare career you may decide to specialize in a particular area such as, for example, diabetes. Again you will develop your knowledge and competence in this role. It may be at this stage that it becomes valuable to move beyond having a sound understanding of the medicines you discuss with patients and the administration of them. Being able to prescribe for your patients will ensure the patient's condition can be managed quickly, safely, and effectively. This will be true for many specialist roles that you may choose. Before embarking on a course to enable you to become a registered prescriber you will

Box 10.1 Useful tips for keeping up to date

- Keep a record of individual interesting experiences involving medicines management
- Take advantage of any training offered, especially those related to medicines management
- Record study days you have attended
- Reflect on study days attended and articles you have read—document them for your CPD portfolio
- Reflect on experiences by discussing with colleagues—again document these as evidence of CPD.

need to be able to assess and diagnose the condition of your patients. Further study may be required and you should seek advice from your manager and pre-scribing course provider.

To conclude this chapter some recently qualified adult nurses suggested the following tips to help compile your continuing professional development portfolio, all of which can be related to the management of medicines (Box 10.1).

Summary

We hope this chapter has identified some of the key components for keeping up to date and provided you with further resources to explore. Now that you have reached the end of the book, you may want to reflect upon it as a whole, and on the journey that you have embarked upon as a nurse.

References

Association for Nurse Prescribers http://anp.org.uk/?s =numbers+of+non+medical+prescribers (accessed 15 November 2012).

See Joint Formulary Committee.

Care Quality Commission (Registration) Regulations (2009). London: HMSO.

Care Quality Commission (2010), *Guidance about compli-ance: Essential Standards of Quality and Safety*. London: CQC.

Davidhizar R (1996). Surviving organizational change. *Health Care Supervisor*, 4; 19–24.

Department of Health (1994), *The Allitt Inquiry: Independent Inquiry Relating to Deaths and Injuries on the Children's Ward at Grantham and Kesteven General Hospital During the Period February to April 1991*. London: TSO.

Department of Health (1998), *A First Class Service. Quality in the New NHS*. London: TSO.

Department of Health (2006a), *Medicines Matters: a guide to mechanisms for the prescribing, supply and administration of medicines*. London: TSO.

Department of Health (2006b), *Standards for Better Health*. London: TSO.

Department of Health (2009), *The Health Act*. Available at: http://www.dh.gov.uk/en/Publicationsandstatistics/Legislation/Actsandbills/DH_093280 (accessed on 4 April 2012).

Health and Social Care Act 2008 (Regulated Activities) Regulations (2010). London: HMSO.

Joint Formulary Committee (2012), *British National Formulary* (64th ed). London: BMJ Group and Pharmaceutical Press.

Latter S, Maben J, Myall M, Courtenay M, Young A, and Dunn N (2005), *An evaluation of extended formulary independent nurse prescribing: executive summary*. Southampton, UK, University of Southampton School of Nursing and Midwifery on behalf of Department of Health, 11; p 5079.

Lewin K (1951), *Field Theory in Social Sciences*. Harper and Row: New York.

Marquis BL, and Houston C (2000), *Leadership Roles and Management Functions in Nursing*, (3rd ed). Philadelphia: Lippincott.

Medicines Act 1968 (c. 67) London: HMSO.

MHRA (2010), *Review of medicines legislation: informal consultation on the provisions for Patient Group Directions and other matters*. Available at: http://www.mhra.gov.uk/home/groups/es-policy/documents/publication/con099711.pdf (accessed on 28 March 2012).

National Patient Safety Agency (2008), Foresight Training Resource Pack 5. *Examples of James Reason's 'Three Bucket' Model*. London: NPSA, available at: http://www.nrls.npsa.nhs.uk/EasySiteWeb/getresource.axd?AssetID=60160&type=full&servicetype=Attachment (accessed 15 November 2010).

NHSBSA, Freedom of information request answers, available at: https://www.ppa.org.uk/foiRequest/foiRequest-Detail.do?bo_id=2132 (accessed 14 November 2010).

Nursing and Midwifery Council (2006), *Standards of Proficiency for Nurse and Midwife Prescribers*. London: NMC.

Nursing and Midwifery Council (2008a), *Standards of Conduct, Performance and Ethics*. London: NMC.

Nursing and Midwifery Council (2008b), *The PREP Handbook*. London: NMC.

Nursing and Midwifery Council (2008c), *Guidance for Continuing Professional Development for Nurse and Midwife Prescribers*. London: NMC.

Nursing and Midwifery Council (2009), *Record Keeping. Guidance for Nurses and Midwives*. London: NMC.

Nursing and Midwifery Council (2010a), *Standards for Medicines Management*. London: NMC.

Nursing and Midwifery Council (2010b) *Essential Skills Clusters*. Available at: http://standards.nmc-uk.org/Documents/Annexe3_%20ESCs_16092010.pdf (accessed on 29 March 2012).

Nursing and Midwifery Council (2010c), *Raising and Escalating Concerns: Guidance for Nurses and Midwives*. London: NMC.

Paediatric Formulary Committee (2012), *BNF for Children* (2012–2013). London: BMJ Group, Pharmaceutical Press, and RCPCH Publications.

Royal College of Nursing (2012), *Clinical Governance*. Available at: http://www.rcn.org.uk/development/practice/clinical_governance (accessed on 10 April 2012).

Scally G, Donaldson LJ (1998). A framework for the analysis of risk and safety in medicines. *BMJ*, 317; 61–65.

Silber MB, (1993). The 'C's' in excellence: Choice and change. *Nursing Management*, 24: 60–62.

The Shipman Inquiry (2004) Fourth Report: The Regulation of Controlled Drugs in the Community: Command Paper Cm 6249. Available at: http://www.shipman-inquiry.org.uk/fourthreport.asp (accessed 4 September 2012).

The Shipman Inquiry (2005) Shipman: The final report. Available at: http://www.shipman-inquiry.org.uk/finalreport.asp (accessed 4 September 2012).

The Times Online (2007) December 7, 2007 Killer nurse Beverly Allitt to serve 30 years. Available at: http://www.timesonline.co.uk/tol/news/uk/crime/article3013216.ece (accessed 18 November 2010).

Glossary

Absolute risk reduction ARR is a way of measuring the size of a difference between two treatments. Put simply, it tells you how much better or worse one treatment is at reducing an outcome in terms of the actual numbers of people who experience the outcome compared with another treatment.

Absorption step the release of medication from its formulation into the body.

Adherence Adherence to medicines is defined as the extent to which the patient's action matches the agreed recommendations.

Administration the act of giving a drug to a patient for them to take at the time that it is given.

Affinity a natural liking for or attraction to something.

Agonist a drug that combines with a receptor to produce a pharmacological action.

Antagonist a drug that combines with a receptor but does not produce a pharmacological action—a blocker.

Bioavailability the extent of a drug that becomes available to its target receptor following administration.

Class effect when all the members of a group of drugs act in the same way, as opposed to the unique action of a single drug.

Competitive antagonism when agonist and antagonist drugs compete for occupation of the same receptor, and the overall result depends upon the concentration of each.

Concordance Partnership approach to medicines management acknowledging equality and using negotiation between the professional and the patient.

Conjugation the act of joining together.

Contraindication factors that increase the risks of using a particular medicine.

Dispensing the provision of drugs or medicines as set out properly on a lawful prescription.

Efficacy the ability of a drug to produce the desired therapeutic effect.

Enzyme inducers An enzyme inducer is a type of drug that increases the metabolic activity of an enzyme either by binding to the enzyme and activating it or by encouraging greater production of it.

Enzyme inhibitors Enzyme inhibitors are molecules that interact in some way with the enzyme to prevent it from working in the normal manner.

First pass metabolism the metabolism of an orally administered drug by the liver resulting in less of the drug reaching the circulation.

Fractional bioavailability the proportion of a dose of medication that reaches the general circulation and is able to act on the body.

Gastroresistant A medicine that is resistant to being broken down in the gastric system.

Hydrophilic Associating freely with water and readily entering aqueous solutions.

Indications The conditions that a medication is intended to treat or the purposes for which it is given.

Intrinsic activity if two drugs occupy the same receptors to the same degree, and one produces a greater response, that drug is said to have higher intrinsic activity.

Irreversible unable to be reversed.

Lipophilic the ability to dissolve or attach to lipids.

Marketing authorization sometimes referred to as a medicines licence; permission from the Medicines and Healthcare products Regulatory Authority to offer a medicine for a particular purpose following consideration of its efficacy and safety.

Mechanism The sequence of steps in a reaction.

Medicinal product Any substance or combination of substances presented for treating or for preventing disease in human beings.

Method of administration The way in which a medicine is given.

Movement part of Lewin's model of change, in which old practice is replaced by the innovative practice.

Non-competitive antagonism When an antagonist prevents a receptor's activity and this cannot be overcome by giving more agonist, this is non-competitive antagonism; usually occurs when the antagonist binds strongly to the receptor, or damages the receptor, or sometimes when it acts at a different site in the opposite way to the agonist so that the net effect is nil.

Number needed to harm The average number of patients who could be treated before an *adverse event* would occur. For example, if the NNH is four, then—on average—for every 4 patients treated, one bad outcome would occur. It is the reciprocal of *absolute risk reduction*. The closer the NNH is to one, the more likely it is that someone on the treatment will experience an adverse event.

For example, if you give a stroke prevention drug to 100 people and two of them experience joint pain, the number needed to harm is 50 (that is, 100 divided by two equals 50).

Number needed to treat The average number of patients who need to be treated to get a positive outcome. For example, if the NNT is four, then 4 patients would have to be treated to ensure one of them gets better. The closer the NNT is to one, the better the treatment.

For example, if you give a stroke prevention drug to 20 people before one stroke is prevented, the number needed to treat is 20.

Odds ratio the ratio, used particularly in case-control studies, estimates the chances of a particular event occurring in one population in relation to its rate of occurrence in another population.

Partial agonist a drug that combines with the relevant receptors but not with the efficiency of an agonist so that its maximum effect is less than an agonist can achieve.

Peer reviewed when something is evaluated by one or more individuals from the same profession, occupation or industry.

Pharmaceutics the science of preparing, using, or dispensing medicines.

Pharmacodynamics the effect that a drug has on the body (how it works).

Pharmacokinetics How the body affects a drug. This includes how the body absorbs, distributes to the site of action, metabolises and excretes the drug.

Prescribing The process of providing a direction, usually written, by an appropriately qualified person, for the preparation and use of a medicine.

Pseudo irreversible some drug-receptor binding is not strictly irreversible, but endures for so long that it is to all intents and purposes not reversible; for example, some poisons will bind to receptors and separate again later, but the untreated patient is likely to die before that happens.

Receptor a molecule on the surface or within a cell that recognizes and binds with specific molecules, producing a specific effect in the cell.

Recognition sites the areas on the receptor where a medicine molecule attaches.

Refreezing part of Lewin's model of change, in which the new practice becomes adopted as the norm.

Relative risk reduction the RRR divides the absolute risk reduction by the original risk that existed.

Selectivity attraction to particular receptors to the exclusion of other receptors; the more selective a medicine is, the more its actions will be limited to the body system it is intended to treat and the less likely it is to cause adverse effects.

Structured search using a database to find information in a systematic way; structured searches may involve linking two desired terms using Boolean operators (AND, OR, NOT) or they may be nested searches, in which the results of each search are then themselves searched using another term.

Supply giving patients medication for them to take over a period of time, for example 25 tablets to take five tablets for five days; medicines legislation uses 'supply' in place of 'sale' to describe the handing over of medicines that cannot legally be sold.

Therapeutic level the concentration of a medicine in the plasma at which it produces a pharmacological effect on the patient.

Toxic level the concentration of a medicine in the plasma at which it produces adverse effects on the patient.

Unfreezing part of Lewin's model of change in which an old practice is shown to need to be discarded and people resistant to change become prepared to adopt a new method.

Unlicensed not having a medicines authorization; distinguish this from 'off licence', when a medicine has an MA but it does not cover the indication for which that medicine is being used.

Index

A

absolute risk reduction (ARR) 106
absorption 44–8
   children 91–2
   entry into tissues 46–7
   older patients 85
   oral drugs 47–8
   rate of 44–5
   site of 45–6
access to medicines 19–20
accountability 2–3, 39–40, 112–14
   clinical governance 113
   ethical implications 112
   legal implications 113
Accountable Officer 6–7, 39
ACE inhibitors 62, 63
aciclovir 63
active failures 35
active transport 46
adherence 133–4, 136, 138
   monitored dosage systems 138,
      139
administration of medicines 7–8,
      10–11, 111–12
   dose see dose calculations
   medication incidents 31–2
   routes 70–81
   timing 31
Adults with Incapacity (Scotland) Act
      (2000) 19
advance directives 19
adverse drug reactions (ADRs)
      63–5
   augmented 64
   bizarre 64
   concordance 137–8
   high-risk groups 82–97
      breastfeeding women 89–90
      children 90–3
      intellectual disability 93–4
      liver impairment 88

   older patients 84–7
   pregnant women 88–9
   renal impairment 88
polypharmacy 94–6
affinity 60
agonists 59
amoxicillin 27
ampicillin, half-life 57
antagonists 59–60
aspirin 4, 50
assault 18
atenolol 49
audit see clinical audit

B

Bandolier 101
best interest 19
bioavailability 77
bisphosphonates 125
blood-brain barrier 49, 78
branded drugs 83–4
breast milk, drugs in 56, 89–90
British National Formulary 10, 39,
      45, 103–5

C

calcium channel blockers 63
capacity 19
Capital and Counties plc v Hampshire
      CC (1997) 25
capsules 71–2
carbamazepine
   drug interactions 30
   enzyme induction 54
   protein binding 51
Cardozo, Benjamin 17
Care Quality Commission 7, 122–3,
      146, 149
Centre for Reviews and
      Dissemination (CRD) 99
change management 146–7

children 90–3
   information for parents 93
   paediatric investigation plan
      (PIP) 91
   paediatric use marketing
      authorization (PUMA) 91
   pharmacokinetics 91–3
Children Act (1989) 90
cimetidine, enzyme inhibition 54
Class A drugs 5
Class B drugs 5
Class C drugs 5
class effects 66
clinical audit 149–50
clinical governance 113–14, 148–9
clinical management plan (CMP) 9
clinical supervision 152
clopidogrel, metabolism 54
Coca-Cola™ 5
cocaine 4, 5
Cochrane Collaboration 100
codeine, pharmacogenetics 58
colestyramine 66
compensation claims 25
competence 38, 40, 152–3
competitive antagonism 61
complementary medicines 67, 119
compliance 133–4, 138
concordance 133–43
   adverse drug reactions 137–8
   challenges to 136
   and consent 136–7
   difficult patients 138–40
   Gibbs' reflective cycle 135
   patient health beliefs 134–6
   within team 136
consent 17–19
   and concordance 136–7
   implied 18
   informed 18
   minors 18–19

continuing professional
        development 144–55
contraindications 30
controlled drugs 4–5, 6
Controlled Drugs Record Card
        (CDRC) 7
creams 79–80
critical appraisal 102–3
Critical Appraisal Skills Programme
        (CASP) 102
critiquing 102–3
cyanocobalamin (vitamin B$_{12}$) 47
cyclo-oxygenase II inhibitors 63
CYP2C9 54
CYP2C19 54
CYP2D6 58
CYP3A4 58
cytochrome enzymes 53
cytotoxic antibiotics 63

D
Dangerous Drugs Act (1920) 4
Dangerous Drugs Act (1967) 4
Defence of the Realm Act (1914) 4
delegation 153–4
dementia 138, 140
diazepam 53
diclofenac 61–2
difficult patients 138–40
diffusion 46
    facilitated 46, 47
digoxin 43, 67
    half-life 57
    protein binding 51
dihydrofolate reductase inhibitors 63
Disability Discrimination Act
        (1995) 20
discharge, preparation for 140–1
dispensing 7–8, 112
    medication incidents 31–2
    one stop 115
    see also prescribing
distribution 48–51
    blood-brain barrier 49
    children 92
    factors affecting 49
    older patients 85–6
    protein binding 49–51

dose calculations 31–2, 128–32
    conversion of metric
        units 127–8
    errors in 128
    intravenous infusions 131
    liquid medicines 130
    ointments 130–1
    SI units 127
    solutions 128
    tablets 128–30
    weight-related doses 131
    see also specific drugs
drugs
    adverse reactions see adverse drug
        reactions
    branded 83–4
    in breast milk 56, 89–90
    controlled 4–5, 6
    dose 31–2, 128–32
    fetal effects 88–9
    generic 83–4
    identification of 31
    see also specific drugs
drug interactions 30, 43, 65–6
    pharmacodynamic 65–6
    pharmacokinetic 66
Drug and Therapeutics Bulletin
        (DTB) 101
drug trolleys 115–16
Dunning, David 38
Duthie Report 115
dysphagia 138

E
E numbers 91
efficacy 60, 61–2
enalapril 53
enemas 74
enteral administration 73–4
enteric coating 45
enzyme induction 54–5
enzyme inhibition 54–5, 62
epidural injection 78–9
Equality Act (2010) 20
erythromycin
    dose 31–2
    drug interactions 30
ethics 112

European Council Directive 2004/27/
        EC 3
evaluations, understanding 105–6
excretion 55–6
    children 92–3
    older patients 87
expert patient programme 141–2
eye drops 80–1
eye ointments 80–1

F
facilitated diffusion 46, 47
Family Law Reform Act (1969) 18
felodipine 66
fentanyl patches 45–6
fetus, drug effects 88–9
fingertip units 80
first pass metabolism 48, 52, 77
fractional bioavailability 48
furosemide (Lasix) 83

G
gastroresistant preparations 45, 72
General Medical Council (GMC) 5
general sales list (GSL) 4
generic drugs 83–4
Gibbs' reflective cycle 135
*Gillick v West Norfolk and
        Wisbech Area Health Authority*
        (1985) 18
glibenclamide 84
gliclazide, dose 32
grapefruit juice, drug interactions 66
guidelines 36–7

H
half-life 56–7
health beliefs of patients 134–6
Health Professions Council (HPC) 2
    Standards of Conduct Performance
        and Ethics 10
Health Technology Assessment
        programme (HTA) 99
herbal medicines 67
HMG CoA reductase inhibitors 63
Human Medicines Regulations
        (2012) 7
hydrophilic drugs 48, 78

I

ibuprofen 61–2
independent prescribers 9
information sources 98–107
  British National Formulary 10, 39,
    45, 103–5
  Internet 101–2
  see also individual sources
informed consent 18
inhalers 75, 125
injections/infusions 75–9
  intradermal 76
  intramuscular 77
  intrathecal and epidural 78–9
  intravenous 77–8
  subcutaneous 76–7
Institute for Healthcare Improvement
    (IHI) 119
insulin 125
intellectual disability 93–4
Internet 101–2
intradermal injection 76
intramuscular injection 77
intrathecal injection 78–9
intravenous infusions 77–8
  dose calculations 131
intrinsic activity 62
irreversible antagonists 61

J

Jowett, Wayne 35

K

keeping up to date 144–55
Kruger, Justin 38
Kruger–Dunning effect 38

L

lansoprazole 66
Lasting Power of
    Attorney (LPA) 19
latent conditions 35
learning disability 139
legal issues
  accountability 113
  rights of patients 17–20
legal roles of health
    professionals 7–10

legislation 3–7
  Adults with Incapacity (Scotland)
    Act (2000) 19
  Children Act (1989) 90
  Dangerous Drugs Acts (1920, 1967) 4
  Defence of the Realm Act (1914) 4
  Disability Discrimination Act
    (1995) 20
  Equality Act (2010) 20
  European Council Directive
    2004/27/EC 3
  Family Law Reform Act (1969) 18
  Human Medicines Regulations
    (2012) 7
  Medicines Act (1968) 3–4
  Mental Capacity Act (2005) 19
  Mental Health Act (1983) 19
  Misuse of Drugs Act (1971) 4–5, 6
  Pharmacy Act (1868) 4
  Shipman Inquiry 5–7, 150
levodopa 43
lipophilic drugs 48, 78
liquid medicines 73
  dose calculations 130
lithium 125
  protein binding 51
liver impairment 88
local intelligence networks (LINs) 6
lock and key hypothesis 58–9
lotions 79–80

M

macrolide antibiotics, enzyme
    inhibition 54
marketing authorization 3
matrix tablets 44
mechanism 144
medication administration record
    (MAR) 116–19, 145
medication errors 134
medication incidents 25–41
  actions leading to 28–32
    dispensing/administration 31–2
    prescriptions 30
    repeat prescriptions 30
    vaccination 28–9
  active failures 35
  frequency 25, 29

  guidelines and protocols 36–7
  latent conditions 35
  near misses 27–8
  never events 28
  Reason's Swiss cheese model 32–5
  reduction of 27
  sources of 26, 27
  system approach 35–6
medicinal products 3
medicine spoons 73
Medicines Act (1968) 3–4, 11
Medicines and Healthcare
    products Regulatory Authority
    (MHRA) 3–4, 39, 90
medicines history 119–21
medicines information centres 101
medicines management 20–3
  components of 110–11
  definitions 109–10
  drug calculations 126–32
  keeping up to date 146–7
  principles 21–2
  record keeping 116–19
  standards 111–12, 121–2
    NMC 15, 22
  systems and procedures 108–25
  see also specific elements
medicines optimization 109
medicines reconciliation 119
Mental Capacity Act (2005) 19
Mental Health Act (1983) 19
metabolism 51–5
  children 92
  cytochrome enzymes 53
  enzyme induction/inhibition 54–5
  first pass 48, 52, 77
  older patients 86–7
  polymorphism 53–4
  prodrugs 53
methotrexate 27, 63, 125
metric units, conversion of 127–8
minors, consent 18–19
Misuse of Drugs Act (1971) 4–5, 6
monitored dosage systems 138, 139
monoamine oxidase inhibitors
    (MAOIs) 43
  enzyme inhibition 54
morphine 4

movement 147
multidisciplinary team 111, 148

N
naloxone 61
naproxen 31
National Health Service *see* NHS
National Institute for Health and
    Clinical Excellence (NICE)
    19–20, 36, 99–100
National Patient Safety Agency
    (NPSA) 26, 109
National Prescribing Centre
    (NPC) 100
National Reporting and Learning
    System (NRLS) 26, 39
National Service Framework for Older
    People 121–2
near misses 27–8
nebulization 74–5
negligence 25
never events 28
NHS Evidence 100
NHS Litigation Authority 25
NHS Service Commissioning Board
    Special Health Authority 26
nicotine
    enzyme induction 54
    patches 45
nifedipine 63
NIHR Evaluation, Trials, and Studies
    Coordinating Centre
    (NETSCC) 99
NMC *see* Nursing and Midwifery
    Council
non-competitive antagonism 61
non-medical prescribers 8–9
non-steroidal anti-inflammatory
    drugs *see* NSAIDs
noradrenaline 59
Northern Ireland, prescription form 14
NSAIDs 43, 63
number needed to harm (NNH) 106
number needed to treat (NNT) 105–6
Nursing and Midwifery Council
    (NMC) 1, 2, 7
    Essential Skills Clusters 15, 20–1
    Guidance for Nursing and
        Midwifery Students 2

Standards for Medicines
    Management 15, 22
Standards of Proficiency for Nurse
    and Midwife Prescribers 8,
    9, 10
Nutt, David 5

O
odds ratio 106
ointments
    dose calculations 130–1
    eye 80–1
    topical 79–80
older patients 84–7
    adverse drug reactions 87
    National Service Framework for
        Older People 121–2
    pharmacodynamics 87
    pharmacokinetics 85–7
omeprazole 53, 66
one stop dispensing 115
opium 4
oral administration 71–3
    absorption 47–8
    gastroresistant preparations 45, 72
    nursing considerations 72–3
    tablets, capsules and pills 71–2
oral syringes 73
Organization of Teratology Information
    Specialists (OTIS) 102
organizations 146
    see also individual organizations
oxycodone 45
    metabolism 52
oxytetracycline 73

P
paediatric investigation plan (PIP) 91
paediatric use marketing
    authorization (PUMA) 91
paracetamol
    dose 32
    prescribing 4
partial agonists 60
pastes 79–80
patients
    access to medicines 19–20
    capacity 19
    consent to treatment 17–19

expert patient programme 141–2
    health beliefs 134–6
    identification of 31
    learning disability 139
    legal rights 17–20
    preparation for discharge 140–1
    visually impaired 140
patient group directions 11, 15, 17, 22,
    113, 145
    students and 15
patient safety 25–41, 148–9
patient specific directions 15–16, 17,
    22, 113
Pemberton, John 5
penicillins 63
pessaries 74
Pharmaceutical Society of Great
    Britain 4
pharmaceutics 43, 70–81
pharmacodynamics 43, 58–63
    older patients 87
pharmacogenetics 57–8
pharmacokinetic drug
    interactions 66
pharmacokinetics 43–4
    absorption 44–8
    children 91–3
    distribution 48–51
    excretion 55–6
    half-life 56–7
    metabolism 51–5
    older patients 85–7
    therapeutic window 57
pharmacology 42–69
Pharmacy Act (1868) 4
pharmacy-only medicines 4
phenobarbital
    enzyme induction 54
    protein binding 51
phenytoin
    enzyme induction 54
    protein binding 51
phocomelia 3
piggy-backing 52
pills 71–2
pinocytosis 46–7
polypharmacy 94–6
    consequences 95
    self-medication 95–6

potassium chloride 27
potency 61–2
povidone-iodine 56
prednisone 53
pregnancy, drugs in 88–9
prescribing 4, 7–8, 112
    errors *see* medication incidents
    independent prescribers 9
    medication incidents 30
    non-medical prescribers 8–9
    private 7
    repeat 30
    supplementary 9–10
prescription-only medicines (POM) 4
prescriptions 11, 12–14
Primary Care Trusts (PCTs) 6
process 144
prodrugs 53
propranolol 49
protein binding 49–51
protocols 36–7
pseudoirreversible antagonists 61

Q

quinolone antibiotics, enzyme
        inhibition 54

R

Reason, James 32
    Swiss cheese model of error
        causation 32–5
    three-bucket model of error
        causation 151–2
receptor blockers 59–60
receptors 58
    antagonism 59–60
    lock and key hypothesis 58–9
    selectivity, affinity and efficacy 60
recognition sites 59
record keeping 116–19
rectal administration 74
refreezing 147
refrigeration of medicines 116
relative risk reduction (RRR) 106
renal impairment 88
repeat prescriptions 30
respiratory tract administration 74–5
responsibility 2–3, 112
revalidation 152–3

reversible antagonists 61
Reye's syndrome 4
rifampicin, enzyme induction 54
risk management 106, 150–1
roles 146
rosuvastatin 53
routes of administration 70–81
    enteral 73–4
    injections and infusions 75–9
    oral 45, 47–8, 71–3
    rectal and vaginal 74
    respiratory 74–5
    topical/transdermal 79–81

S

St John's wort 67
salbutamol 48
    structure 59
Sale of Goods Act 3
saw palmetto 67
Scotland, prescription form 13
Scottish Intercollegiate Guidelines
        Network (SIGN) 100
Scottish Medicines
        Consortium 100
selectivity 60
serious untoward incidents
        (SUIs) 38–9
shaving 80
Shipman, Harold 5, 150
Shipman Inquiry 5–7, 150
SI units 127
side-effects *see* adverse drug
        reactions
significant event analysis (SEA) 38
sildenafil 63
skills specialization 154
slow release preparations 44
sodium valproate, protein
        binding 51
solutions of drugs 128
standard operating procedures
        (SOPs) 37
standards 111–12, 121–2
    NMC 15, 22
statins 63
steroids 124–5
    inhalers 75
stock cupboards 115–16

stock management 114–15
storage of medicines 115–16
students, and patient group
        directions 15
subcutaneous injection 76–7
sublingual administration 73
substituted judgement 19
supplementary prescribing 9–10
supply of medicines 7–8, 111–12
suppositories 74
suxamethonium 27
    pharmacogenetics 57
Swiss cheese model of error
        causation 32–5
systems and procedures 108–25
    need for 109
    see also medicines management;
        and specific elements

T

tablets 71–2
    crushers 73
    cutters 72
    dose calculations 128–30
talking labels 140
teratogenicity 88–9
terbutaline 59
thalidomide 3
theophylline, therapeutic
        window 57
therapeutic level 57
therapeutic window 57
three-bucket model of error
        causation 151–2
Toft, Brian 35, 38
topical administration 79–81
topoisomerase II inhibitors 63
toxic level 57
transdermal administration 79–81
transdermal patches 45
transpeptidase inhibitors 63
transport inhibitors 62–3
Treaty of Versailles 4

U

unfreezing 147
United Kingdom Medicines Information
        service (UKMi) 100–1
uptake inhibitors 62–3

V

vaccination, medication
    incidents 28–9
vaginal administration 74
vancomycin 45
vascular access device (VAD) 78
vicarious liability 20
vincristine 35
visually impaired patients 140

vitamin B_{12} (cyanocobalamin) 47
vitamin K epoxide reductase
    inhibitors 63
voltage-gated calcium channels
    (VGCCs) 63

W

warfarin 50, 63, 125
weight-related doses 131

workforce issues 151–2
working with others *see*
    multidisciplinary
    team
World Association of Medical Editors
    (WAME) 102

Y

yellow card system 39